Cycle to the Moon

Cycle to the Moon
© Veronika Sophia Robinson
© Illustrated by Susan Merrick
ISBN 978-0-9575371-4-9
Published by Starflower Press, Summer Solstice 2014. www.starflowerpress.com
British Library Cataloguing in Publication Data. A catalogue record for this book is available from the British Library.

Also by the same author:
Fields of Lavender (poetry) 1991, out of print.
The Compassionate Years: history of the Royal New Zealand Society for the Protection of Animals, RNZSPCA 1993
The Drinks Are On Me: everything your mother never told you about breastfeeding (First edition published by Art of Change 2007) (Second edition by Starflower Press 2008)
Allattare Secondo Natura (Italian translation of The Drinks Are On Me 2009) published by Terra Nuova www.terranuovaedizioni.it
The Birthkeepers: reclaiming an ancient tradition (Starflower Press 2008)
Life Without School: the quiet revolution (Starflower Press 2010), co-authored by Paul, Bethany and Eliza Robinson
The Nurtured Family: ten threads of nurturing to weave through family life (Starflower Press 2011)
Natural Approaches to Healing Adrenal Fatigue (Starflower Press 2011)
Stretch Marks: selected articles from The Mother magazine 2002 – 2009, co-edited with Paul Robinson (Starflower Press)
The Mystic Cookfire: the sacred art of creating food for friends and family (more than 260 vegetarian recipes) (Starflower Press 2011)
The Blessingway: creating a beautiful Blessingway ceremony (Starflower Press 2012)
Baby Names Inspired by Mother Nature (Starflower Press 2012)

Fiction
Mosaic 2013
Bluey's Cafe 2013
Blue Jeans (illustrated children's book) 2014

Other illustrated publications by Susan Merrick:
What a Lovely Sound! Written by Starr Meneely 2013
Blue Jeans, written by Veronika Sophia Robinson 2014

Cycle to the Moon

celebrating the menstrual trinity

menarche
menstruation
menopause

By Veronika Sophia Robinson
Illustrated by Susan Merrick

Starflower Press

Dedication

For Susan Merrick ~ How do I even begin to express my overwhelming gratitude for your artwork, and for bringing this book to life with your passion and enthusiasm?
Thank you so much for believing in women.
For my soul systers, you know who you are. I love that our cycles are in sync, regardless of how many mountains or oceans separate us.
For my daughters, Bethany and Eliza.
You have grown into gorgeous women. I love you.
Never doubt for a minute how incredibly proud I am of both of you.
My mother, Angelikah, for teaching me that Moontime is natural.
And for my beloved, Paul: you are my one true home. Always.
Veronika

For the women in my life,
and for Noni, who told me to 'just keep drawing'.
Susan x

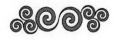

Let's Cycle Together!

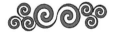

It's been a long journey, the journey home. How far along the road am I? From the little girl with flowing hair, taught at every turn to hate her specialness, her power, her female core - to the woman, mother, lover who begins furtively to honour her woman's soul image. I remember the little girl - I now hold her in my heart (her wounding is my healing). She sits with me now. In her I taste the first blood and the first flows. I remember my father's distaste and horror at our femaleness... He tried to turn us girls into boys.

Sally,
Cycle to the Moon workshop participant.

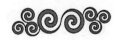

Welcome

Welcome to *Cycle to the Moon*. May this journal give you a sacred and safe place to discover and celebrate your femininity. May it be a friend throughout your menstrual life, and may the pages upon which you write offer a special gift to share with your daughters and granddaughters.

It can be used regardless of where you are on the menstrual trinity (menarche: first blood; menstruation and motherhood; menopause: last blood) or where you are on your cycle. Let it be your mirror: a reflection of how you see yourself. All you'll need is a pen and some colours: paint, crayons or pencils ~ and quiet, reflective time. All the information and activities are offered as support and loving guidance. If you need medical help, seek it.

I wrote the first draft of *Cycle to the Moon* in 1998. I'd been menstruating for fourteen years. I had birthed two daughters; experienced two miscarriages (I would later have another two); had stress-related haemorrhaging; and lactation amenorrhoea (absence of bleeding) for a total of thirty two months. At that point, my periods had been easy and gentle. As at publication, 2014, I am a woman who has been menstruating for just over thirty years. I have endured (and healed) debilitating menstrual migraines. I have learnt so much about my body, the Moon, and the way to reconnect with myself. It is only now that I can see why it took so long for this journal to be published. I had to have a more substantial menstrual history! For years I had been waiting for the right artist to collaborate with. How lovely that the wonderful Susan Merrick arrived in my life as the first whispers of menopause call to me from the night sky. It is with excitement that I walk, confidently and, I have to admit, rather damn excitedly, towards this next chapter of my journey as a woman: the wise crone.

I was sixteen when I went on the contraceptive pill. The synthetic hormones played havoc with me. I went from size eight to eighteen (Australian dress size) in a matter of six months. I came off the pill, and have never used chemical contraception again. In my

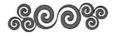

early twenties, I was sexually harassed by my employer. I ended up haemorrhaging for months, so disconnected was I from my body. My body and my mind were were in denial about my femininity and sexuality, and this expressed in such a violent blood flow. I now feel deeply connected to Nature, my life and the Universe. My periods are once again gentle and enjoyable, and I cycle with the Moon every 29.5 days. I enjoy charting my cycle. As a child, my mother would write the word *tage* on the calendar for several days each month. Tage is the German word for period. It makes me smile that I too write *tage* when noting the days I bleed.

If you are new to the Menstrual Trinity - welcome. May your cycle always, and in all ways, be a pleasure. I wish for you that it be a time of deep, inner renewal. If you are now experiencing menopause, bless you. Thank you for bringing your womanly wisdom to the world. Please allow the Moon to still guide you even after your last flows have ended. You can use Moon maps and other techniques in this book to remind yourself of the lunar rhythm. Every aspect of your life is beating to the great lunar pulse.

This book was conceived while I was breastfeeding my youngest daughter, Eliza. At the time, I was not menstruating, and thought it was a bit strange to feel the inspiration to write a book on it! However, between that time of living on the sunny east coast of Australia and then moving to the cold of northern England, I have visually held the women of the world in my mind. I initially put together the final pages of the first draft of this book, snuggled by the open fire, with my toddlers playing 'mummies ' nearby. Their presence reminded me of all the cycles of our lives. I prepare for publication, many years later, as my daughters stand at the edge of the nest, preparing to leave home in the next couple of years. My body is preparing for menopause, gently and easily. I am walking ahead towards this new part of my life consciously and with excitement.

This book features quotes from women who attended my workshops *Sacred Cycle* and *Cycle to the Moon*. I've met women who honestly and openly shared their experiences of what it was to be a woman in modern times. Most felt wrapped beneath a heavy, dirty blanket of fear, shame, pain and hurt. *Sacred Cycle* gave them the courage to let go; the

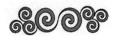

confidence to buy sanitary products at the supermarket without feeling shamed to hide them beneath the groceries; the freedom to walk with their heads held high, and glad to be a woman regardless of where they were on the menstrual trinity: menarche, menstruation or menopause. Together we cried, and together we laughed.

One of the greatest gifts my mother gave me was the belief that having my period was natural. I was never brainwashed with the common Western negativity of "The Curse". In fact, I felt somewhat cheated when all my school friends had their period and I had to wait until I was 16 before my cycle started. To me, it signified the start of womanhood. I was ready! It is only now that I understand the truth: I wasn't a late bloomer. I was a young woman blessed to grow up deep in the heart of the countryside, well away from artificial night lights. I ate a plant-based diet, free from animal hormones, and the synthentic hormones and antibiotics readily found in meat. These two things have a huge impact on when a girl begins menstruating.

My best friend at school was Cherry. On the day of her first period, I had raced excitedly to her house because we'd planned to go swimming in the dam. Her dad met me at the door and told me she was sick and couldn't come swimming. I was disappointed. When I found out later that she had her period, I felt like her father had lied to me. "She's not sick," I thought. "She's just bleeding. Of course she can go swimming!" In an amazing coincidence, as I was typing the above paragraph, Cherry phoned me. Amazing, because it was our first contact in ten years. I loved that, despite the miles and years between us, we were still 'connected' in such a profound way. During our chat we talked about the often silly ideas our parents pass on to us. She said, "Do you remember the first day I got my period? My Dad made out I had a sickness. When I asked Mum when it would happen again, she said in 'four weeks'. That's all she ever told me about my period!"

Another woman said the first day she got her period her mother sent her to school with a huge bag of sanitary pads. She wondered, "Am I supposed to carry these around all day?" Unfortunately, for many of us, our mothers had grown up with such fear and shame that it was a lot easier for them to say nothing at all! "The Curse", and other negative

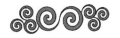

ideas associated with the menstrual cycle, need to be banished. Too many young girls are growing up with the belief that this normal, natural event is dirty and something to be ashamed of. Why? The power of women's blood, the power of Moon week, is something to be honoured. It is a cleansing in the deepest sense. A time to let go, and a time of renewal.

Cycle to the Moon has been written to celebrate the cycles in your life. Through these pages you will learn ideas, techniques and thoughts to help you understand the power and beauty within your body. You will find guidelines to bring you back in tune with your body and with the Moon.

There was a time when women governed the world, not in a dominating sense, but rather as gentle mothers who nurtured their young, precious children. One day, some men started to rebel against women's gentle power, and began to rape, torture and condemn. Women were burnt at the stake. The world was turned upside down. For so long women had held civilisation together beautifully with their innate understanding of the Moon, the seasons and the Earth's rhythm. They understood the healing power of herbs, prayer, of rites of passage. Women were respected for their wisdom during menstruation. The communities of long ago relied on women's menstruation and their timing with the Moon as the base for accounting, mathematics, music and even architecture. The foundation of civilisation relied upon our cycle! Religion, science and agriculture were also based upon our menstrual cycle. Our blood was not only used for ceremony but to capture animals and to fertilise fields.

The overturn of a matriarchal society saw the invention of Satan and a masculine God. Because men had had no power in this society, the only thing left was fear. So they had to convince other men to turn on women. According to *Conversations with God* by Neale Donald Walsche, the understanding of women having a direct line to the Goddess was so powerful that men had no choice but to invent a devil to 'counteract the unlimited goodness of the Great Mother'. And so, the myth began. By using such thinking, men started questioning if women really were superior. Over many, many years, the innate

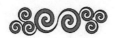

love and compassion of women was overtaken by a male hunger for power. The jealous God was born, and the wrathful one. We humans have turned myth into what many people call reality, and, in turn, many women have lost their sense of living in tune with the Universe.

So the world changed: women learnt to distrust their bodies. In fact, they felt ashamed. They forgot their power to birth beautifully and easily. Their periods became painful. Menopause was a trial. Bleeding women were considered 'evil'. We, as women, need to reclaim our power. It is our responsibility. But unlike the patriarchal domination which currently rules the world, we need to gently guide Earth and her people back into harmony. We can start by honouring and nurturing our own bodies and that of our sisters and daughters. From here, the love will ripple out into the world and back again. We must share this with our daughters. We must wake up. It is time. To cycle to the Moon gives us a deep understanding of the Universe. A balanced planet is once again achievable through the intuition and strength of the menstruating and menopausal woman. Our body, mind and soul are linked. Reclaiming the magic of menstruation will heal us.

This journal is designed to help you reclaim your menstrual power. To understand ourselves more fully, and why we culturally deny our menstrual power, we first have to understand our Herstory.

Our menstruation is our honesty.

It tells us what the world denies.

It is a mirror of our diet, emotions, beliefs, cellular memories,

dreams and the world we live in.

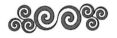

wild moon woman
you were not made to be tame.
you are an earthquake shaking loose
everything that is not soul.
shake, woman, shake.

~ Elyse Morgan

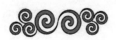

The Ancestresses

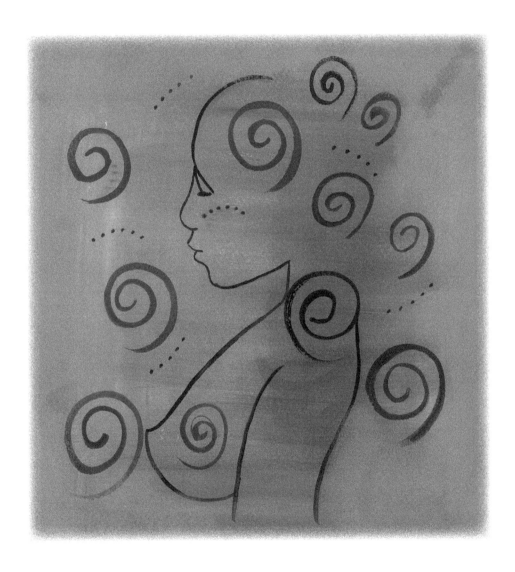

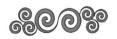

It may seem as if we've always lived under patriarchal rule, but archaeologists are often discovering cave paintings and other evidences of a Goddess-based world. In cultures around the world, the Great Goddess is known by different names. What defined these cultures is that they all lived in accord with Nature: recognising the cyclical nature of the Earth, the Moon, and their own bodies. Sexuality was sacred. These women were guardians of the land, revered Nature, and passed their land, possessions and knowledge down the maternal family line. The Bronze and Iron ages which began about 3,000 years before the birth of Christ, saw nomadic warriors come from Northern Europe and Central Asia into the peaceful Goddess cultures. In their path they left a trail of destruction and disempowerment. Women were raped, slaughtered, exploited; and children were sold as slaves.

Archaeologists have evidence showing large-scale destruction of the Goddess culture long before man-made religion had its effect. Church and property laws changed. Anyone who dared speak out about this was burnt. The all-loving, compassionate, mother-image of the Goddess was changed to one of darkness and evil and one to be feared. Men now owned women. The Goddess teachings were denounced, and the female mysteries of birth and cycles were forced into hiding. Over five and a half centuries *at least nine million people were killed* in what was known as the Witch Hunts. Witches included children, psychics, midwives and wise women. These were people who understood the sacred nature of sex, herbs, and midwifery. Those who survived the torture, branding and rape were burned. Witchcraft came to include many things. In 1593, a jailer discovered a clitoris, and never having seen one before, thought it was a Devil's teat: proof that the witch was guilty. She was burnt.

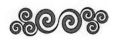

In 1593, a jailer discovered a clitoris,
and never having seen one before,
thought it was a Devil's teat:
proof that the witch was guilty.

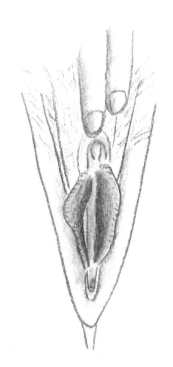

We now know that the clitoris has one purpose: pleasure.

Using your non-dominant writing hand, write whatever comes to you regarding the parental or cultural messages you were given (or not given!) on menstruation. What images were you given about women's bodies? What messages, verbally or through body language, were you given about your body?

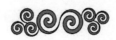

Myths, Memories and Legends

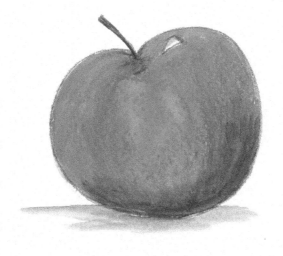

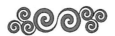

Women haven't always had a menstrual cycle synchronised to the Moon. Our move away from oestrus (seasonal cycling to the Sun) and into bleeding monthly, rather than seasonally, gives us the choice when to have sex. This was our evolution.

In the Bible, this is what Eve shared with Adam *(from Adamah, which means 'bloody' clay)*. Eve plucked the apple of menstruation, known biblically as the *tree of life*. We now choose when to have sex rather than having it forced upon us by Nature. This also means we can have sex for pleasure, and not just procreation. This was not original sin but the ultimate liberation. Thanks, Eve! Somehow, though, this got twisted in the translation from Hebrew to Greek to English! The word 'sin' is an old archery term that was called out when the arrow missed the bullseye. It literally meant to 'miss the mark'.

Many ancient myths, legends and stories tell of our fall from grace. One theory suggests that the change occurred when we moved away from eating a diet largely of raw fruit and leaves: the chemicals in these tropical foods triggered our happy hormones. Where once we lived in harmony with Nature and ourselves, we moved away from divine consciousness into a state of ego-driven function. The state of bliss we had in the tropical forests, and our pure diet, meant we had no need for a period as regular as the one we have now. There was, in essence, no need to release toxins from our body.

Native American Indian women had a dreamtime in which they all gathered together in their Moon Lodge. Together they would cycle to the Dark Moon. Being such an intuitive time, everyone in the village would gather together. The men honoured these women and would come to ask questions. They nurtured them by preparing food and drinks. Within the teepee-like Moon Lodges were areas of thick green moss to sit on. It was here the blood was collected. At the end of the week it was buried in the land as part of the ceremony. Interestingly enough, the men must have felt like they were missing out on something, as it was from the Moon Lodge that the men's Sweat Lodge came into being.

Women in what became known as Rhodesia built themselves special menstrual huts for seclusion.

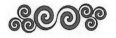

Tibetan women would use a few drops of their menstrual blood, mixed with food, to feed the man they desired to be with for life. They believed this would bind them together.

In Tantra, Dakini means the 'red goddess'. That is, menstruation. Women from the Shetland Islands would lay themselves in the moonlight. In Papua New Guinea, the Trobriand Islanders spend a whole day on a puberty ritual. It's a very social occasion. The celebration includes the men chewing betel nuts so they can spit red juice on the newly menstruating girl. The red is symbolic of the bleeding time. They call menstruation 'the Moon's embrace'. Culturally, an Amazonian girl can expect six months of seclusion when she starts her cycle. Her diet consists of ants and termites. At the end of the six months, she is given a ritual bath. Women from the Torres Straits say the halo around the Moon is her blood. Apache Indians hold a four-day dance called Sunrise when a girl starts menstruation. She wears an abalone shell across her forehead to symbolise the changing woman. Members of her tribe shower her with bright-yellow pollen.

The early Christian Church considered the blood of menstruation to be 'wasted babies', hence the mass killing of witches for 'killing babies'. Nine million women were burnt for knowing their woman-craft. That is to say, they understood their dreams, used herbs, and celebrated the process of menstruation. Witch means *woman*. Their craft, woman-craft, was, quite simply, understanding the mysteries of life. Ironically, some early Christians held sacraments where the worshippers consumed a mix of menstrual blood and semen.

The Taoist practice is for men to take red yin juice (menstrual blood). They believe that a woman's vagina leads to immortality. The vagina is considered the Mysterious Gateway.

The field workers of Germany called menstruation 'the Moon'. Women from India practise their woman-craft by moonlight. Traditionally, Brazilian girls begin their cycle with three months of seclusion, and then a three-day party.

Much washing and dressing occurs in the New to the Moon ceremony of the Ghana tribe, Dipo. First the girl is adorned with beads. She is then taken off for a ritual bath in the river,

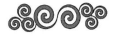

for it is here she meets the river's spirit. Finally, she has raffia ropes put around her neck. The Aboriginals of Australia state that the Moon tames women, and that women are under her spell. In France, the bleeding time is called 'le moment de la lune'.

The Mohave Indians give special attention to the dreams of a young woman at menarche. They represent her spiritual ability and a prophecy of her life's path. She is urged to share them with a tribe elder. Sri Lankan and southern Indian girls celebrate their first period by eating raw egg which has been flavoured with ginger oil. They sit on a bed of banana leaves. This is followed by a bath in milk. The family comes together for an end of the day feast. Congo women call their period *the Moon*.

In New Zealand, the Maori say the Moon is a menstrual goddess, and that our relationship to her is our real marriage. They talk of Moon sickness in the way some other women talk of love sickness.

Early people carved marks on bones to represent the Moon's phases, and then coloured red ochre for their bleeding time. Aristotle was known to have recorded the 'new Moon' menstruation of women.

The legend of the Dagon goes that Mother Earth's skirt was stained with her menstrual blood. Red soil, probably. A human woman found it and became Queen of the Land. The skirt was stolen by a man who then claimed rulership!

Ancient Egyptians used menstrual blood for healing, as an ointment, and in the making of medicine. In Cambodia, secluding a girl for several months when she reached menarche, enabled her to draw on her psychic senses. When she returned to the light a great celebration was held.

The menstrual cycle was used as a calendar by the Romans, Moslems, Indians and Babylonians. They associated menstruation with the Moon. South American Indians believed all humans were created from Moon blood.

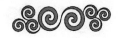

Menstrual mythology refers to menstrual blood as life-giving, as opposed to our modern cultural belief of it being 'waste' blood.

Hindus would bathe in menstrual blood, believing it would increase their vitality. Some kings believed that drinking menstrual blood would lead to immortality. From Hawaiians to South African bushmen we find menstrual myths, stories and legends.

In almost all languages, the words Moon and menstrual are the same, similar or from the same root word.

All cultures hold rich beliefs about our bleeding time. This makes us vastly different to other animals, which, to our knowledge, do not ritualise menstruation.

Women created seclusion to nurture themselves during the time that their five senses were reduced (menstruation), and their sixth sense (intuition) was increased. This area, known as the third eye, is where the pineal gland is situated. Men enforced this seclusion out of fear. Our fears pass through the generations like a poison. There never used to be fear associated with our Moon time. We can consciously create the wisdom of our foremothers, and celebrate our cycle openly and honestly.

Some women regularly go out during their bleeding time and release blood onto the earth as a way of connecting. One woman in New Zealand, who was building a new home, collected her Moon blood in a jar for four cycles. At the end of each cycle, she buried it in the land at one of the four corners of her new home. This was her way of dedicating and honouring herself and her new living space. Another woman in England recalls a past-life memory when she had her first period. She was greatly honoured by everyone. The blood was kept in a small jar as ointment, and was used to bring healing to her family. I remember the story a Canadian lady told me. She'd always had a very difficult time with her periods. This lasted many years, until she made peace with her body. Now she hardly notices when she has her period. Each lunar month she puts her Moon blood into the earth at the four corners of her home.

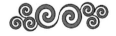

Once upon a time there was a young girl who lived in a beautiful valley. Although she was young, she was, in fact, nearly a woman. Each day she would walk the valley, collecting herbs and flowers to bring back to the Moon Hut. This was the special place where all the women of the valley would gather during the Dark Moon. The young girl had now been invited to join the women.

Her body was changing. Where once she had tiny nipples on her chest, she was now growing malleable breasts. Her once bare, naked pubic area, was now as soft as moss with black downy hair. Her hips were round. It happened one day as she was standing on the cliff top overlooking the valley and singing a beautiful song. An inner stirring had drawn her there. And as she stood, the warmth of women's power ran down her legs. As she looked downward, drops of deep, red blood touched the earth. And the girl knew, she had become a woman!

Her name was La Luna. She stood for some time at the cliff top as Maiden of the Valley before returning to her mother and foremothers. A great celebration was held that night in the Moon Hut. There was much music, dancing, and feasting on fine fruits. The women brushed her hair, and washed her feet. They sang her songs and told her stories. La Luna was welcomed into womanhood. She was told how her precious body would one day be a fine vessel for new life, and that a spirit baby would one day fill her womb. The women each shared a way in which she could care for herself and prepare her body using herbs and flowers.

The blood that had stained La Luna's skirt was used as a 'welcoming' flag for strangers that came to the valley. And from that day on, La Luna's Valley became known as the Red River Valley.

Create a legend you would like to share with your young women friends and family about the wonder of a woman's cycle.

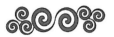

I am a woman.
I can make life and nurture it...but where is my man?
Where is the man who will love me for being a WOMAN?

Ruth, Cycle to the Moon workshop participant

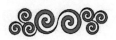

Include a photograph or drawing of yourself at the age you began menstruation.
What do you remember about this day? What were you doing? Who did you tell?
Was it a time of celebration or secrets? Were you honoured?

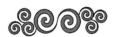

How did you feel when reading Herstory?
What gifts can you bring to menstruation (yours, and that of other women) which will help to heal the cellular memory of our Herstory?

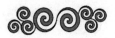

The Menstrual Calendar

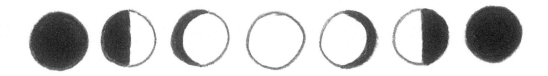

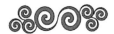

If I could be given a gift from my mother about my cycle,
it would be a ceremony to welcome me to womanhood.
We would go outside in the dark and light a red candle
to thank the goddess for our bonding.
We would drink red wine and pour wine upon the earth as a blessing.

Ruth,
Cycle to the Moon workshop participant

Menstruation is your body's own calendar. Essentially, in a healthy female, it is a cycle of about 29.5 days (the same as the lunar cycle, whereby it takes that amount of time from one full Moon to the next) dictated by various hormones in the woman's body. It begins at puberty, and continues through to menopause, generally in a woman's fifties. It occurs each lunar month unless interrupted by the contraceptive pill, stress (including crossing international date lines, poor nutrition, extreme exercise), ill health, pregnancy or breastfeeding.

Given the number of years for which we have a menstrual cycle, it is worth understanding how it happens to us and how we can 'enjoy' our bleeding. It affects us not only physically, but emotionally, mentally and spiritually; even if we're not consciously aware of it. Our cycle begins on day one of our period, when a follicle-stimulating hormone (FSH) is released by the pituitary gland. This hormone makes its way from the brain, through the bloodstream, to the ovaries. Inside the ovaries, it stimulates the follicles. Their job is to prepare a number of eggs for ovulation. As this is happening, oestrogen is released by the ovaries. This causes the cervix to lift and become soft. It also increases 'sperm friendly' mucus. The lining of the womb makes itself ready for the possibility of fertilisation. The level of oestrogen rises. The oestrogen signals back to the pituitary gland, which then sends Lutenising Hormone to release the ripest egg from a follicle in the ovary. The chosen egg goes into the fallopian tube to wait for fertilisation. This is the process we know as ovulation, usually occurring at about day fourteen of the cycle. Back at the ovary, there

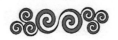

is now an empty follicle. It is called the Corpus Luteum. This temporary, small gland releases small amounts of oestrogen. This signals to the cervix to close up and harden to a state of infertility. The mucus also dries up. While the Corpus Luteum does this, it also releases progesterone to thicken the endometrium (womb lining). This is to prepare for the egg which is travelling from the fallopian tube to the uterus. It also tells the ovaries to stop releasing eggs. Should pregnancy occur, that is, the egg successfully implants into the womb lining, the level of progesterone will rise until after childbirth. On the other hand, if there is no fertilisation, the Corpus Luteum dies; the production of hormones stops. The womb lining breaks down and is released as our menstrual blood. And so this approximately 29-day cycle begins again. A balance in the level of hormones secreted is required for regular menstruation.

Create a handmade Moon map for recording phases and biorhythms.

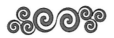

Listen to your body talking. What is she saying? Are you aware of how technology and modern living affect your wondrous body temple? Listen. Listen. Listen. What do you need? When was the last time you walked barefoot on Mother Earth, or slept under the stars? Nature always offers the best medicine: air, sunshine, water, real foods and the right environment to exercise.

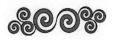

Create your own Moon Calendar

Either use a new calendar for each month or leave enough space and use the same one for 13 Moons, and watch the spiral grow. This way you can more easily see your own ebb and flow.

An effective way of preparing yourself for possible PMT is by drinking a lot more water two weeks before your period, and adding a lot of water foods like lettuce, watermelon and cucumber to your diet. Increase foods rich in the B-complex vitamins, too. If you want to enjoy an easy cycle, you have to cut out sugar and processed foods. Have them as rare 'treats', not as staples.

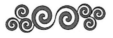

Moon Mandala

A mandala is a wonderful tool for aligning oneself with the Moon and with Mother Earth. Essentially it is a circle with points. By drawing this wheeled cross and putting in the four Moon phases, we can consciously feel the rhythm of our lunar beat. You can write your cycle phases next to the appropriate Moon phases. That is, ovulation, post-ovulation, menstruation and pre-ovulation.

Draw or create one each month from feathers, stones, leaves, twigs, pine cones, shells or maybe even one from fruit. Allow your innermost creativity to come out. Be voluptuous, passionate, childlike, ripe, full, creative. A mandala can be intensely private or an intimate community affair. Watch how it changes with the seasons and how you change with your growing awareness of cycles.

A moveable mandala, like a bracelet, can usually be purchased from marketplaces. Wearing one is a constant reminder of the circles of our life.

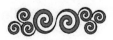

The Moon Calendar (full Moon to full Moon) is twenty nine and a half days, the same as the healthy woman's menstrual cycle. The Gregorian calender does not fit into our cyclical way of living. Let's change it. Obtain a Mayan Dreamspell Calendar or create your own Moon Calendar.

Why not wear a red ribbon around your wrist when you have your period? It's a great visual reminder to slow down and honour your flow. Some women wear a red bracelet during their period. This lets friends and family know: *be gentle with me, my body is on sabbatical.*

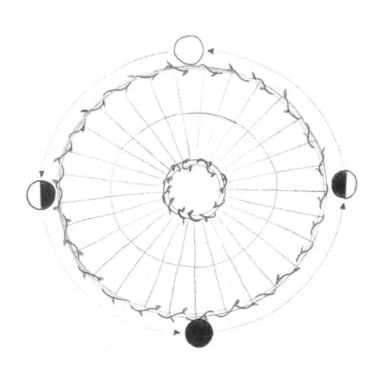

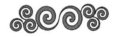

What have I observed by recording my cycle? How can I help myself? What do I need?
Is there anything I'm not asking for? What is stopping me?
How differently might I feel if I had my needs met?

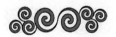

Sisters of the Moon
rituals to support the moontime

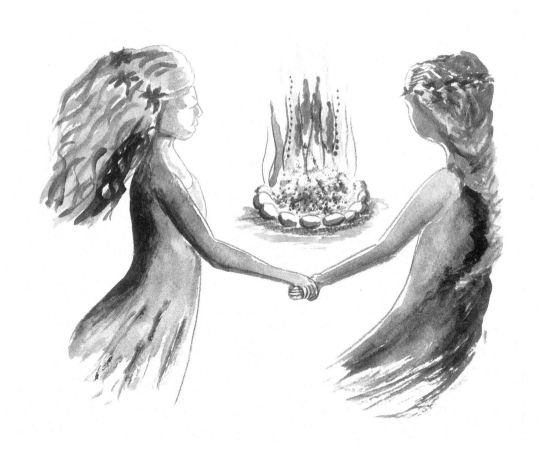

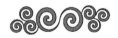

Labyrinth

Labyrinths have been used since ancient times to evoke a sense of calm and peace. Use this finger labyrinth (starting from the large red flower bud), and mindfully follow the vine until you have completed the journey. Ask yourself what it is you most need. Relax and breathe deeply.

Seven paths,
seven portals,
seven veils,
seven layers,
winding round towards the soul.
Finding Self in bones and blood,
safe, contained,
with space to wonder,
entering the flow.

~ Karen Schluter

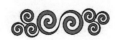

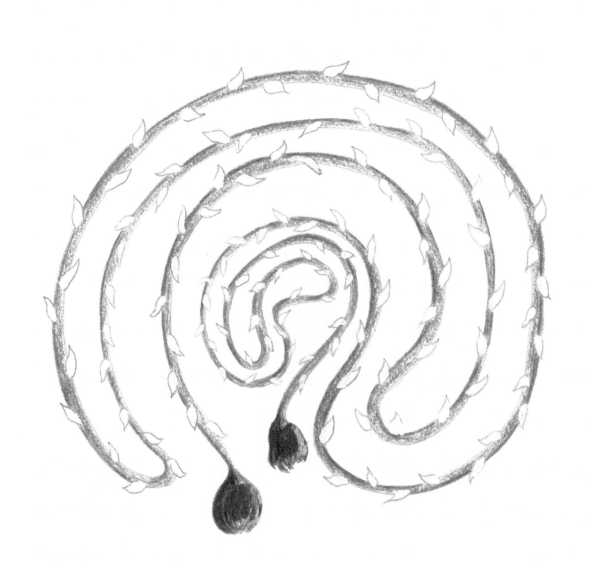

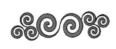

The Red Box

On the eve of my elder daughter's first period, I presented her with a red box. Together we'd been collecting special items to put inside. This included a book of menstrual legends, soothing herb teas, a mandala, red fabrics and cushions, cloth pads, jewellery, candles, a Moon calendar, and other special items, like a goddess bookmark. When her period arrived, her younger sister made a special celebratory meal of red foods: red pepper and tomato soup, a red salad of tomatoes and radishes, and we had pink ginger drink. Creating a box of treasured items is something your daughter will always remember. You can include anything you feel that celebrates the cycles and femininity. It might be a Goddess pendant, cloths, scarfs, paper, a mirror, Moon charts and calendars, herbs, such as dried sage, red raspberry leaf tea, red candles, ruby or garnet gem stones, red underwear, red ribbons.

Another way to create the Red Box is to gather the contents in secret, and present it to your daughter during her menarche ceremony. You can do this on your own, or with contributions from the women in your Red Tent community.

When my younger daughter had her first period, we shared this occasion, just the two of us, by reading menstrual stories and creating a Red Tent in her bedroom. We decorated it in red scarves and fabrics, red cushions, we lit candles, and burned incense and played music. I had collected red flowers, and arranged her hair in a new style. By candlelight, I welcomed my beautiful daughter across the cusp of womanhood. It was a private occasion, as befits her personality.

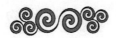

The Red Tent

The original meaning of sabbath was menstrual seclusion. This is what our ancestresses did: they bled together on the dark of the Moon, and nurtured each other in the privacy of a Red Tent. This rapidly growing worldwide movement to reclaim the Red Tent is a visible rising of the collective energy to celebrate the spiritual practice of our wisdom around menstruation.

Like our ancestresses, we come to the Red Tent to bleed, to find sacred space during our Moon time. This could be a shared space with other women in the community, or it could be your bedroom, or sacred place in the garden, or Nature. It could even be a virtual Red Tent where you meet other women online to share your experience.

It is common to bleed at the same time as your best friend or women you share a living space with. When we consciously come together with other menstruating women, such as in the Red Tent, we're giving ourselves permission to be free of the concerns of life: permission to be free to dream, care, relax and nurture ourselves. Reclaiming the ancestral Red Tent means that we no longer deny menstruation. We consciously celebrate our bleeding time, and our bodies.

The Red Tent is a beautiful way to celebrate menarche. This first blood is a rite of passage, and to be held and encircled by the women in your community in this way is a memory that will last a lifetime.

The only way to change our culture is to change the practices within it. Each and every one of them is in our hands. We are powerful, and we can heal the sacred feminine individually and collectively.

The Red Tent is a symbol. It is a reminder that we need to retreat for some of our menstruation. We are women, not machines. We're not designed to work around the clock, seven days a week.

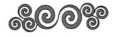

Have you ever experienced a Red Tent? If not, create one in your mind. Who is there? What does it look like? How does it nourish you? How does the idea of this women's community feel to you? Is this something you would like to create in your life?

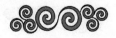

Even without a community Red Tent, you can create space. It might be snuggling up in bed and writing in your journal, or taking a candlelit bath (without the kids!), or perhaps lying on your back in the woods and feeling Mother Earth beneath your skin.

The simple truth is that menstruation is a mirror of your life. If you're not honouring your body through healthy food choices; ample hydration (three litres of water a day); rest; playtime; calmly managing stressful events; positive thoughts; creativity and sleep; then it will show up in your menstrual cycle. However, your hormones will come to call, and they will *demand* that you rest. You might try and quiet them down with headache tablets or something pharmaceutical for cramps, but they will keep talking to you (even if it takes twenty years), until you get the message. If you don't honour your body during the menstrual years, you are highly like to suffer when you reach menopause.

As we hold the hands of our young sisters when they cross the menstrual threshold, we would be wise to remember that their experience of this cycle will affect them throughout their childbearing years and into menopause. There's a red thread which weaves through these major themes of our life. Every moment is connected. Whatever we have learned and integrated benefits not only us, but the culture.

The Red Tent, symbolic or physical, is also an altar upon which we can teach our daughters and young sisters the truth about the disposable sanitary products industry: it contributes countless chemicals and toxins to this beautiful Earth, taking hundreds of years to break down; pesticides harm the fields and rivers, and block our drains, pollute our seas, and infiltrate landfills. How easily we get caught in the endless cycle of purchasing these products. However, upon the altar of the sacred feminine, we can share the revelation that there is another way, a holistic way: reusable soft cloth pads, sponges, Moon cups. Together, you can stitch pads which will last years and years. *See the pattern on page 154 to make your own cloth pads.*

As a menstruating woman releases her blood, she can give it to the herbs and trees in her garden. As she offers it up to the Earth, she can make prayers with her blood and dedicate it to any of her intentions.

An actual conversation between mother and daughter

Mother: *"What are you thinking about?"*
Daughter, aged five: *"I'm thinking about when I get my first period. Could we have a party to celebrate? Could you buy me some grapes to eat? And could I sit on the moss to bleed like women used to long ago?"*

Conversation between sisters
as they're folding up mother's washable menstrual pads

Daughter, aged 3.5 years: *"I want Moon pads like Mummy's ones when I grow up."*
Daughter, aged 5.5 years: *"I won't need Moon pads unless I live in a cold country because I am going to sit on the moss when I have my Moon time."*

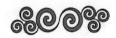

The Maiden's Initiation

I remember menarche clearly. I had just turned sixteen years old, and was on a holiday on the other side of Australia, some 2,000 kilometres from my home. I was staying with my mother's sister; my aunty Helga. When I told her my first period had arrived, she was embarrassed. I, on the other hand, was excited! My friends had all been bleeding for years. My aunty asked me what my mother would say, and how she'd deal with it. I replied "She'd be honest and direct." It seems funny to recollect and realise I was the one educating my aunty about the normality of the female cycle.

These days, sixteen would be considered a late time to start menarche, based on the statistics of city girls. I was a child of Nature, raised on a plant-based diet free from animal hormones and antibiotics, and lived in the heart of the countryside a long way from street lights.

It is never too early to share menstruation with your daughters and sons. I explained to my daughters, when they were aged two and four, that: *the bleeding doesn't hurt.* They even raced to get me a cloth pad from my bedroom drawer! A four-year-old child can grasp the story of the ovary making an egg. If the egg doesn't meet up with the seed (sperm from Dad during the 'bouncy cuddle') that there is no baby, and it becomes menstrual blood. This early learning becomes very matter of fact, and teaches children things the way Nature intended rather than being kept in the closet until puberty. Right from early on, they can learn the Moon's phases by comparing it with the shape of a banana or apple. Don't be afraid to take them out into the night and share the wonder of this great luminary which sails through the sky over a quarter of a million miles away.

Where possible, a father should be an important part of his daughter's menarche. He could honour it through a gift, such as a red rose, red necklace or red dress. He needs to acknowledge his daughter's sexuality and to show her that he is aware of her growing into a woman. How different our culture would be if more young women were celebrated by their fathers in this way.

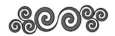

Cut an apple in half to reveal the star pattern. I showed my daughters that they looked the same with hands and arms apart, jumping for joy! Let your daughters know that we have the benefit of this fruit of knowledge. Eve didn't lead us into sin, she liberated us! She knew the truth about that apple! Oh yes, it was the fruit of all knowledge alright. Eve wasn't trying to be 'naughty' or disobedient, or to leave us a legacy of perpetual misery and sin. She was showing us the way!

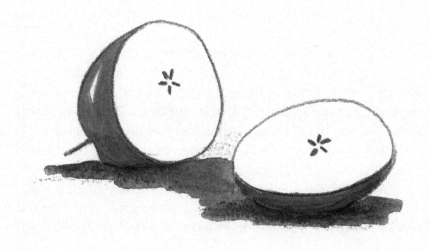

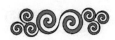

Dear Maiden, Welcome to the Moontime. Congratulations! How do you feel about your first blood? What stories have you been told? How would you like to experience your cycle?

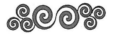

Create your dream Red Box. What do you find inside? What do these items mean to you? Who has put these items in there? What else would you like to find inside? If you have never received a Red Box, make one for yourself. It's never too late to honour the inner Maiden. Fill it with nourishing items, and bring it out each Moon week in celebration of your amazing body.

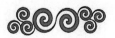

First Blood Ceremony

As a celebrant, I love to officiate ceremonies. If you wish to create a First Blood ceremony, follow this framework. Always begin a ritual by creating a sacred space. There is no place for modern technology in a ceremony, so ask guests to turn off their phones. Place a sign on the door asking visitors not to disturb.

Before guests arrive, create a peaceful ambience by lighting candles. White ones are perfect for this occasion. Burn incense, such as rose or jasmine. Play music that is gentle and inviting. Perhaps it is something the Maiden has chosen herself? Another option is to have the guests gently hum or chant.

Before the ceremony, you will have set up a small altar containing gifts or items that are meaningful for the Maiden, such as a statue, picture, or objects from Mother Earth. There may be flowers or a dish with red dye or henna.

A circle can be created using red scarves, rope, henna, wool or other natural fibres. As the celebrant, you can either have this in place before guests arrive, or unwind it around the circle once the ceremony begins. If you have dried sage, this would be a good time to smudge the circle (also known as the Medicine Wheel). Alternatively, sprigs of lavender are beautiful to scatter around the ceremonial area. You might like to sprinkle rose petals over the guests or make a pathway into the circle for the Maiden to enter.

Have the young Maiden sit in the centre of the circle or next to the altar. As the ceremony begins, invite her to put her bare feet into a bowl of warm water with fresh herbs or flowers inside.

Some New Moon traditions involve a large bowl filled with cornmeal. The Maiden is asked to step into it, and leave her footprints. Women in the circle step forward, light a candle, and place it into the cornmeal. This is symbolic of her journey on this beautiful Earth.

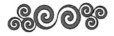

Just like in other women-only ceremonies that I officiate, I invite each woman to introduce herself in this way: I am Veronika. I am the daughter of Angelikah, and the granddaughter of Leiselotte and Minna-Marie.

This would be a good time to share in a song.

Ancient Mother
Ancient mother, I hear you calling
Ancient mother, I hear your song
Ancient mother, I hear your laughter
Ancient mother, I taste your tears

From the *Blessingway Songs* CD, by Copperwoman

As each woman introduces herself and her foremothers, she promises to offer guidance and friendship to the Maiden on her journey through all the cycles.

Afterwards, the Maiden introduces herself. She, too, lights a candle. She accepts the blessings of the circle.

This is now the time to adorn the Maiden. Henna or earth-based body paints (see resource section) are a lovely way to do this. Or you can make her a flower crown. I did this for one of my daughters, using dark-red flowers, and it was truly beautiful.

Gifts can be given at this time, including the Red Box. For example, jewellery, underwear, books. When women share their gifts, it is helpful to the ritual if they say why they are giving that particular item to the Maiden.

Include songs, stories of first blood, positive words, and poetry. With all ceremonies, symbolism is rich with meaning and speaks a thousand words.

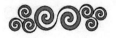

At the end of the ceremony, the women form two lines, with their arms raised to create an archway. The Maiden takes a toy or item from her childhood as she stands at the entrance. A Wise Crone calls to her: *Who is approaching this pathway?*
The Maiden says her name.

The Wise Crone (or celebrant, if there are no wise crones in attendance) says: *Dear Maiden (name), it is time to let go of your childhood so that you can join our circle. When you are ready, leave your childhood at the entrance.*

The women stand in silence as she makes her walk. When she reaches the end, the Wise Crone (or celebrant) marks it symbolically by throwing rose petals, or ringing a bell.

A final song or prayer is shared, and then the circle gathers for red food and drinks. You might like to choose a song, such as this one:

Circle Surrounding

There's a circle surrounding the circle we are in (*three times*)
The Angels, Beings of Light
Calling in the Angels, to be by our side
Knowing, when we call them
Their light is here to guide our way
Their light is here to guide.

From the *Blessingway Songs* CD, by Copperwoman

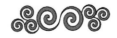

Colour

Candles are an important part of a ceremony. Throughout *Cycle to the Moon*, the artist, Susan Merrick, has used white, red and black. These colours are symbolic of the deep and sacred feminine. White is for the virgin, the Maiden. It represents purity and innocence. With red, we are symbolically painting the fertile, child-bearing woman. Red is the colour of our blood. It is our passion, our creativity, our vibrancy. It says we're *alive!* Black is the crone. The wise woman. She is a lady of experience. Her life comes from her heart. Our culture may use black for grief and mourning, but it is also used for introspection.

Altar

There are so many lovely symbols which can find their way onto an altar: seashells, clay, matches, rocks, feathers, gems, wood, seeds, eggs, nuts. If there is a wise woman in the family who has a special piece of jewellery to share, this is a lovely place to put it. Images of the Moon also have a special place here: The waxing Moon, for the Maiden. The full Moon, for the Mother, and the waning Moon, for the Crone.

Special, magic, clever, wonderful, I love, peaceful, high, we work, bodies work, amazing, normal, painless, quiet, shameless, shameful, cold-shouldered, ignored, hurtful, powerful but secret, ashamed to show feelings, emotions, laughed at, embarrassed, hiding from everyone, symptoms and feelings and needs, Sacred, celebrations for being a woman or hidden from the world by ashamed relatives...compressed, suppressed by everyone you come into contact with.

Anna, New to the Moon, 16 years old, extract from the Sacred Cycle Workshop about the associations she had with periods.

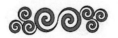

The Moon Woman's Medicine Bag

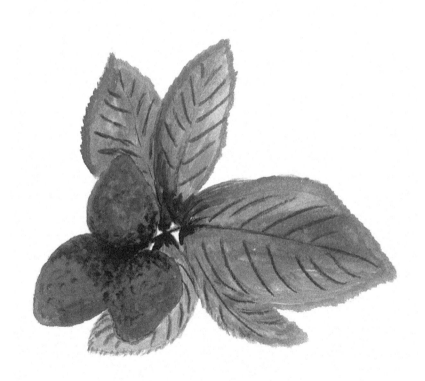

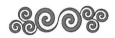

Your diet is going to be reflected in the way your body cycles. There is no getting around this fact: you are what you eat and drink. It has been found that women who eat low on the food chain and have nutrient-rich diets have easier, often pain-free, periods. The word period came from the 'dot' of blood (as in a full stop) in the underwear of African women who were transported to America as slaves. Their diet comprised unprocessed foods, so their body had no excess toxins to clear out each month. A scant period doesn't necessarily mean a deficient diet.

Women who eat nutritionally balanced diets are unlikely to feel bloated or have headaches. Their period may, in fact, only last for a day or two. Some women who have a diet high in raw food, that is 70 - 90% raw fruit and vegetables, barely know they're having a period. Regardless of whether you eat meat or are vegan, your diet needs to be nutrient-rich, and filled with plenty of foods of all colours, in as close to their natural state as possible.

Adding foods rich in calcium and Vitamin-B complex reduces premenstrual tendencies. It may take many weeks or months for the Vitamin B to help you, depending on how deficient you are. The B-complex vitamins require a diet rich in protein to work best. If you are struggling with PMT, I advise finding a good-quality supplement to kick-start your healing. A peri-menopausal woman, for example, would find a supplement (such as Biocare's AD206) beneficial. I highly recommend transdermal magnesium (spraying magnesium on your skin several times a day), as the body consumes magnesium rapidly when we're under any sort of stress.

Try high-quality vegetable proteins for easier digestion. Signs of calcium deficiency include insomnia, depression, irritability, headaches and nervousness. You will also need vitamin D (at least twenty minutes of sunlight a day), and magnesium for calcium absorption. Fifty to 100 years ago, women didn't start their periods until their late teens. Now it is common for girls as young as nine and ten to start their cycle. As mentioned, one reason is that the meat, poultry and dairy products of today's diet are so high in hormones that it is accelerating the start of the menstrual cycle. The other reason is artificial light, and living our lives as if it were normal to work or play through the night.

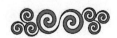

Japanese women don't even have a word for menopause. They don't appear to suffer the way Western women do. It is no coincidence that they have a diet high in soy products, which contain natural oestrogen. It is also interesting that their incidence of breast cancer is rare due to the iodine-rich diet (seaweeds).

Remember to include iron-rich foods in your diet, such as kale. Don't be tempted by synthetic iron tablets. If you need extra iron support, opt for Floradix, a gentle tonic made from the aqueous extracts of spinach, a variety of fruits, herbs and honey. Alternatively, have one to two tablespoons of organic, unsulphured, blackstrap molasses a day. Try it as a nightcap mixed with creamy organic soy or rice milk. It is delicious hot or cold. Or try Spatone's iron-rich water. You could make a daily smoothie of spinach leaves, banana, avocado, coconut oil, cinnamon and a little maple syrup. Nettle tea is invaluable for raising iron levels. None of these natural forms of iron causes constipation like iron tablets do. Ideally, it is best to supplement with a complete wholefood to balance any vitamin and mineral deficiencies. A quick test to check your iron levels is to pull down your lower eyelid. The inside should be red or bright pink. If it's pale or white, then you need to address the situation quickly. You'll be feeling exhausted and run down. Chocolate and caffeine inhibit iron absorption. Once we begin our lives as menstruating women, we need to be particularly mindful of consuming plenty of iron-rich foods.

Iodine is vital for *every* hormonal receptor in the body. Breasts need *100 times more* iodine than the thyroid. Many countries, such as Australia, have iodine-deficient soils. So, if you don't eat fish, ensure you regularly eat seaweed or have kelp. Iodine deficiency can lead to menstrual migraines as well as an inability to absorb vitamin B12. Please note: *women with large breasts need even more iodine*. If you suspect iodine deficiency, don't rely on a standard doctor's test. Get it done privately through a reputable laboratory, because even a marginal deficiency (which won't show on a doctor's test) can leave you debilitated. Symptoms include: dry skin, unexplained weight gain and inability to lose it, snoring, inability to tolerate the cold, dry hair, hair falling out, menstrual migraines, fatigue. If you need iodine, avoid synthetic versions, and stick to kelp or other seaweeds. You can't overdose on natural iodine. Your body will excrete unnecessary iodine through your urine. Cranberries are also rich in iodine.

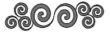

If you're on the contraceptive pill, be aware that synthetic hormones play hell with the body, and suppress a natural process. The consequences may take years to surface. There are several pills in a pack which are taken to produce a period, but these are merely sugar pills. The bleeding is a false period as such, known as withdrawal bleeding. This is ironic, as it gives women a sense of normality around their cycle.

Women who follow a natural diet, that is, they eat primarily plant-based foods, find their periods to be light. In fact, a comprehensive study of these women, and women in indigenous cultures who eat such foods, shows clearly that the menstrual flow of women is, by nature, meant to be light, easy and painless. So, include more fresh raw fruits and vegetables in your daily meals.

Despite the widespread use of cooking throughout the world's cultures, the human body is not designed for such food. It is true that we have learnt to adapt, to a certain degree, but as soon as processed or cooked foods enter the mouth, white blood cells throughout the body race to the intestines in defence! Millions of years of ancestral knowledge live within our cells, so each time this happens, these immune defenders are off doing other work and not the job they should be doing. So, include as much raw food as you feel comfortable eating.

The vagina and its excretions (mucus and blood) are a mirror of the foods and non foods (that is, junk) we put into our body.

Here are a few nutritious Goddess salads to rev you up!

**Make a bright red salad: red onion (sliced), red peppers and red cherry tomatoes. Drizzle with a little balsamic vinegar.

**Grate one raw beetroot. Cut an orange into cubes. Grate a little organic orange zest, and add half a clove of crushed garlic. Mix together. Enjoy!

**Combine two grated carrots, one chopped orange, a tablespoon of desiccated coconut, a handful of sultanas, and a cup of sprouted chickpeas.

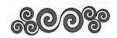

** Combine one orange capsicum/pepper, half a red cabbage finely shredded, a large, handful of homegrown sprouts (chickpeas/lentils/mung) and a handful of chopped curly parsley.

Vegetables should be your primary food source, as they're rich in vitamins and minerals. Aim to eat plenty of root vegetables and leafy greens.

Choose brown rice, corn, oats, rye, millet, buckwheat, quinoa, amaranth, lentils, kidney beans, azuki beans, chick peas, haricot beans, lima beans, black-eyed beans, black beans, split peas, seeds and nuts. Include fresh fruits in your diet, as they are an important source of fibre and vitamins. Avoid unhealthy fats, and use virgin olive oil, avocado, coconut oil or hempseed oils.

Miso, almonds and quinoa are good sources of protein, and help fight fatigue. Despite myths about food-combining and protein, a full complement of protein is obtained over the course of a day by eating a variety of foods.

Seaweeds are rich in minerals, vitamins and amino acids. Include them in your daily diet. They include kelp, dulse, spirulina, chlorella, Irish moss, bladderwrack, blue-green algae, Iceland moss, and red marine algae. They are considered amongst the best and most nutritious foods you can eat.

Iron-rich foods include: kale, yellow dock root, burdock root, dandelion root, nettles, elderberries, red raspberry leaf, rooibos, and mullein leaf. You can also eat parsley, greens, chives, spinach, and blackstrap molasses (unsulphured). Try drinking dandelion and burdock tea each day.

Calcium is found in almonds, sesame seeds, comfrey root, oatstraw and red raspberry leaf. It is found in all leafy greens.

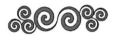

Essences

Essences are vibrational medicines that work on the subtle bodies. They are made from the energetic material of plants, animals and gemstones. These gentle essences are non-addictive and completely safe. You place a few drops under the tongue or in a glass of water four times a day. They can also be administered by adding to bath water, or placing drops on your wrist or temple. Unlike homeopathy, you don't need years of study to find a remedy. The following outline is all you need. Select whichever emotional state most suits where you're at. It is possible to select more than one remedy. Up to five may be chosen. For a dosage remedy, place two drops of essence into a 25ml dropper bottle and fill with equal parts brandy and still mineral water. Take four drops, four times a day. Don't keep a made-up remedy for more than three weeks. The following Bach Flower Remedies may help at various times during your cycle.

Cerato - unsure of self; repeatedly seeks advice of others
Gentian - depression from known cause; pessimism
Hornbeam - inability to cope with daily tasks; lack of strength
Walnut - sensitivity to outside influences
Holly - jealousy and suspicion/feelings of revenge. PMT
Rock Rose - extreme fear/panic/terror
Mimulus - fear of known things
Cherry Plum - desperate and suicidal/fears own actions. PMT
Aspen - anxiety and apprehension
Red Chestnut - irrational anxieties
Chicory - self-indulgent and self pity/demands attention
Impatiens - impatience and irritability. PMT
Olive - complete physical and mental exhaustion
Mustard - deep gloom and depression
Oak - for the effects of endurance when under pressure
Crab Apple - obsession with cleanliness; self condemnation. Helps to deal with shame/sexual trauma. Also for toxicity associated with menopause.
Star of Bethlehem - clearing childhood trauma.

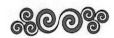

Australian Bush Flower Essences produce *Rose of Raphael essence* which assists female fertility and sexuality.

Other essences which may benefit women in the menstrual trinity:

Amazon Waterlily - receptivity to creating sacred space
Self-Heal - empowerment through clarity of healing direction. Negative Feelings *[Menopause]*
Sunflower - identity crisis. *[menopause]*
Zinnia - enjoyment of life; celebration *[menopause]*; opening up to play
Borage - grief at the end of menopause, especially if childless
Bougainvillia - awareness of self. (Hawaiian Tropical Flower Essences)
Chamomile - meditation; moodiness (Flower Essence Services)
St John's Wort - dreams/nightmares *[Menarche]*
Fairy Duster - finding balance for one's own needs (Desert Alchemy)
Macrozamia - empowering women (Living Essences); awareness and balance of femininity. Freedom from the negativity of incest/negative sexual experiences

Sister Moon Flower Essence Oils
These anointing oils enhance and help expand your most important relationship: the one with yourself.

Celebrating Women's Beauty (for a strong sense of self belief)
Women's Healing Lodge (gateway into the safe, warm womb of the sacred healing places within you)
Sisters of the Moon Time (Empowerment/Rites of Passage/Creation/Gestation/Nurturing)

All essences are available from Healing Orchids.
See resources.

The Herb Garden

I can't emphasise enough that a healthy, clean and wholefood diet is the most important step you can take to have easy and gentle periods. It can take some time to undo the damage caused from a nutritionally inadequate diet, sugar, caffeine, processed foods, or periods of extreme or ongoing stress. In the meantime, herbs may help you.

These herbs can make your flow easier: maca, black cohosh, blue cohosh, dong quai, mugwort, red raspberry leaf, wild yam root, squawvine, false unicorn, chaste tree berries, lycii fruit, red clover tops, liquorice root, sarsaparilla, and angelica. You should consider herbs and any other natural supplement as a support to a conscious way of eating and drinking, not a replacement.

To ease cramping: beth or birth root, crampbark, fennel seed, anise seed, and wild yam root.

For menstrual headaches: white willow bark, black willow bark, feverfew, meadowsweet, birch bark, wood betony, wild lettuce, peppermint, wintergreen, and woodruff.

To calm the nerves: nerve root or lady's slipper, kava kava, jatamansi, valerian root, lavender flower, passionflower, hops, skullcap, chamomile, and linden flower.

To boost energy: ginseng (all species), ashwagandha, schizandra berries, jiwanti, yerba mate, green tea, suma, codonopsis bark, kola or bissey nut, and guarana seed.

If your breasts are sore during menstruation, try massaging (in a base of olive, coconut or almond oil): fennel seed oil, clary sage, grapefruit-peel oil, and rosemary, saw palmetto berries, honeysuckle flower, red raspberry leaf, red clover tops, yew tips, poke root, wild indigo, and red root. Tender breasts are a sign of iodine deficiency.

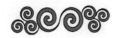

Natural Helpers

Craniosacral therapy can help ease menstrual-related problems. Our bodies are living tissues which need to breathe and move. The cranial rhythm, which moves throughout our being, can be described as subtle rhythmic impulses. A therapist is able to move these by reading the body with his/her hands, that is, by listening with their fingers for any patterns of congestion.

The movement involves the central nervous system, the cerebrospinal fluid and surrounding tissues and bones, including the skull. The natural sense of order of the body, when disturbed, results in the cranial motion becoming congested or restricted. Balance and integrity can be maintained through cranial therapy. The gentle touch revitalises the tissues. It is a non-invasive therapy.

Homoeopathy is based on "like curing like". The remedies come from the essence of plants, animals and minerals, and latterly the environment. Because it is a complex science, it is recommended you consult a qualified practitioner. If you're unable to find one, the following suggestions may be helpful. Do not take remedies within an hour of using strong-smelling substances such as aromatherapy oils, peppermint, coffee or toothpaste.

Belladonna: for excessive menstrual cramping pain.
Magnesia Phos: for pain that is relieved by pressure or warmth.
Chamomilla: for menstrual discomfort associated with irritability and moodiness, particularly if pain is aggravated by anger.
Pulsatilla: for the woman who is moody and depressed. If you have no thirst, and open air relieves your discomfort, this remedy is for you.

Do some nutritional research of your own. Which foods are rich in Vitamin B, iron, zinc and calcium? Create some delicious recipes you can use to boost your intake, particularly two weeks before menstruating, but ideally every day. Invite your friends around to share a meal. The B-complex vitamins reduce anxiety, fluid retention and mood swings.

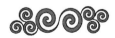

Take selenium and iodine for tender breasts. You can meet your selenium needs with just a couple of Brazil nuts each day. Headaches? Vitamin E and iodine. Anxious or depressed? Calcium and magnesium deficiency are probable. Ironically, the products you turn to for comfort - *coffee, sugar, chocolate, alcohol* - are the ones which will do you the most harm! Weaning yourself from these items will bring great benefits.

Sacred Sabbatical

It's important to retreat, and honour our menstrual mysteries. We *need* the dark phase of our body's cycle for regeneration, dreams, healing, sacred sexuality, meditation and inspiration. Our yin-yang cycle of ovulation and menstruation is needed for optimal health. It's important to recognise that we're never unproductive even if it appears, on the surface, that we're still, quiet and contemplative. This is a rich time of rejuvenation. In our 24/7 culture, menstruation is no longer recognised as 'down time'.

As consciously menstruating women, we can liberate ourselves from this grip by knowing that we don't always have to be busy. Menstruation is a time to let go of ideas, beliefs, projects and plans. This then allows us access to our creative world, and here we learn to live life consciously. We have no reason, other than cultural, to act as if we're fertile all the time. By trusting that it is not only okay, but vital, to have 'me' time, is to be fully present and available to ourselves. When we ignore our body's needs, it will react. We give this reaction many names, commonly:

Premenstrual syndrome (tension)
Depression
Cramps
Menstrual headaches/migraines
Mood swings
Cravings

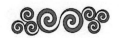

We must turn the menstrual tide and bring ourselves back to shore. Nurturing ourselves is vital. Why is this so hard for us to do? Who told us it was selfish?

Ritual and ceremony help to bring us back home. There are many ways of tuning into your menstrual cycle. The most common is to track your ovulation and menstruation against the Moon's cycle. Each day, write down how you feel. Note the phases of the Moon, and the zodiac sign.

Soldier's Moon: Aries
This is the sign of action and pioneering. We can feel impulsive and even angry when the Moon transits Aries. Watch for cuts, bites, burns and stings.

Builder's Moon: Taurus
I love to bake and spend time in the kitchen when the Moon is in Taurus. This is the sign of creature comforts and stability.

Scribe's Moon: Gemini
Watch communication pick up when the Moon is in jittery Gemini! This is a good time to phone friends or walk around your local area and catch up with the neighbours.

Shield-father's Moon: Cancer
Ruled by the Moon, the sign of Cancer teaches us about nurture and nourishment, and taking care of people, plants and pets. This is the sign of home.

King's Moon: Leo
Leo loves a stage! The Moon here can find us wanting an audience, and to perform. It's a particularly creative sign.

Weaver's Moon: Virgo
Virgo likes routine, ritual and cleanliness. The best use of this phase is for getting your house and health in order. It is a good time for mentoring: passing on knowledge or skills to another person.

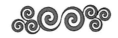

Ambassador's Moon: Libra
Time for mediation and having friends for dinner. This is the sign of beauty and socialisation, fairness and balance.

Witch's Moon: Scorpio
Scorpio invites us into the depths so we can transform ourselves. You may feel your emotions more deeply than usual with this transit.

Philosopher's Moon: Sagittarius
Freedom is the keyword here, both physically and mentally. Sagittarius wants us to explore new horizons.

Grandfather's Moon: Capricorn
This is the time to put structures in place, and solidify your ideas.

Apostle's Moon: Aquarius
Humanity is the keyword of this Moon. A time to think about your place in the world, and the part you play, and how to leave it a better place.

Moon of the Angels of Mercy: Pisces
Be mindful of your boundaries. Pisces is compassionate, but this energy can soon have us swamped in other people's emotions.

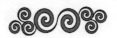

Phases of the Moon

The Moon is constantly waxing and waning. Become aware of her cycles, and notice how your emotions ebb and flow.

The *New Moon* rises at dawn and sets at sunset. Because of the brightness of the Sun, you won't actually see the Moon on this day. The Moon rises a little bit later each night, so you'll see a sliver of Moon in a day or two, just after sunset, hanging low in the western sky.

The *Crescent Moon* is the second phase of the cycle, noticable by the dim outline of the Full Moon. It reminds us that we're heading towards fulfillment. You'll see it after sunset.

The *First Quarter* Moon rises in the east at noon, and sets in the west at midnight. At sunset, you'll find it above the southern horizon, half light, half dark. It is only visible for the first half of the night.

The *Gibbous Moon* rises in the east, mid to late afternoon. You can see it clearly, even before sunset. It will set around three in the morning, and is almost full.

The *Full Moon* shines the whole night through. It rises in the east at sunset, and sets in the west at dawn.

The *Disseminating Moon* rises mid-evening, and sets mid-morning: big, bold and beautiful.

The *Last Quarter* rises after midnight, and sets around noon.

The *Balsamic Moon* rises after three in the morning, and sets mid-afternoon, its light growing thinner and thinner reminds us that the New Moon is near.

Observe the phases of the Moon for at least a few months, if not for the rest of your life, making a note of your feelings and the daily events of your life.

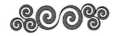

Topics to write about:

Mood

Creativity levels

Mucus/blood secretion

Energy levels

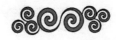

Describe your period. How many days do you bleed for? What colour is your blood? Go beyond blood red. What does it *really* look like? Is it dark pink (showing low vitamin B status), muddy brown, crimson red? What does it feel like to touch? How does it smell? What is the consistency like? Is it thin or thick and clotty? Touch your blood. Get to understand your body. What does it remind you of? Don't be afraid. The blood is from the core of you! How do you feel about your flow? If you don't bleed on day four of your cycle, but bleed again on day five, this is a sign of adrenal fatigue.

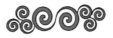

Draw two maps of your body. One during your bleeding time and one at ovulation. Explore both images. Imagine safe hands exploring your innermost regions. What are they saying? What can you learn about yourself and your needs?

My Menstruating Body

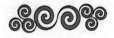

My Ovulating Body

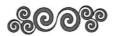

Water

Water is widely used in antenatal care for pain relief. Try it when you're uncomfortable, whether from bloating or cramping, or just plain irritable and need time to yourself. Add a few drops of essential oil to your bath to enhance the experience.

Floatation Therapy (also known as Restricted Environmental Stimulation Therapy) is one of the most effective means of stress relief and relaxation available. Science validates its benefits. The gravity-free environment brings you as close as you are ever likely to be to an experience of complete weightlessness. I can't recommend it highly enough for bringing calm into your life, and lowering cortisol levels. If your periods bring you pain, increase your vitamin B levels, and enjoy floatation for quick absorption of magnesium.

Floating creates homeostasis and harmony in the body, rests the five senses, balances both hemispheres of the brain, the body's skeletal and muscular system, and balances the mind, body and spirit.

Research shows that floating measurably reduces blood pressure and heart rate whilst lowering the levels of stress-related chemicals in the body. Physically, it offers relief from inflammation of the joints, lower back pain, tired aching muscles, insomnia and stress, and it's very beneficial for boosting circulation. Not dissimilar to the Dead Sea, which enables the individual to float effortlessly on its surface, the water in the floatation tank is heated to skin temperature. It is virtually impossible to distinguish between parts of the body that are in contact with the water and those that aren't, thus creating the illusion of floating in air.

It can be used to alleviate depression, addictions, fears, phobias, learning and emotional issues, as it induces the release of endorphins (the body's natural opiates) and has proven to be excellent for accelerated learning, powerful affirmations, self-hypnosis, meditation and visualisation for health and well-being.

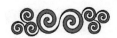

Smell

Our sense of smell is deep rooted. Even a newborn baby can find his mother's breast from the faint smell of her milk. There are many essential oils available on the market. Make sure you only buy 100% pure essential oil from reputable distributors. Here are a few ideas to get you started. Tea tree, clove, rosemary and cinnamon are excellent for antibacterial and antiviral protection. Lemon, bergamot, lavender, rose otto, jasmine and geranium enhance our performance abilities. Cardamom, juniper, rosemary, pine, bergamot and grapefruit are ideal if you need to be alert. Try a few drops in massage oil, using almond or grapeseed oil as a base. Alternatively, add it to an aromatherapy burner, or a couple of drops in a water sprayer to freshen up a room.

Movement

Movement is vital to life. Without it, we seize up. Even if you're not sporty, and particularly if you lead a sedentary lifestyle, try to incorporate some simple and gentle stretching/ strengthening exercises into your day. Why not try yoga, swimming, bellydancing or walking 30-40 minutes about four times a week? Or you could join your local gym.

Colour

Colour is life. Imagine our world without it. Colour is everywhere. As a therapy, it has been taught and practised for thousands of years. Red-based colours tend to produce tension in our body (raising blood pressure) and lift energy, while the blue range lowers blood pressure.Colour can be consciously increased in our life in many ways. Through the use of lamps (coloured bulbs or ones covered with coloured cellophane); fabric (the clothes we wear, and furnishings in our home); solarised water (*see note below) and colourful foods. We can practise colour visualisation and colour breathing. Ninety percent of light enters our body through our eyes. Natural sunlight provides the full spectrum of colour that our bodies need. People who live through deep, dark winters are deprived of this nourishment, and often suffer Seasonal Affective Disorder.

When we have been upset emotionally or spiritually, or have been physically unwell or hurt, an imbalance is created in our aura. An aura is the interacting colour energy patterns

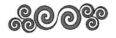

around our body. It is not normally visible to the human eye. Visualising colour allows us to release years of negative thinking, which ages us. *To make solarised water, fill a glass container with pure water, and place it in the sunshine (either outside or on a sunny window sill) for a couple of hours. Leave it all day if cloudy. Either use a coloured glass or wrap coloured cellophane around a clear glass. Drink the water throughout the day. This is an easy and wonderful way of absorbing the full spectrum of sunlight.

Each colour has its own quality. Close your eyes, and focus on each one. Write down what your sense is of that colour, and if you need more of it in your life. Think about colours in terms of food, clothing, decorations, Nature.

Red - *vitality, willpower, strength and sexuality, groundedness.*

Orange - *fun, happiness and joy.*

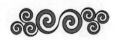

Yellow - *digestion, increases intellect, mental alertness.*

Green - *balance, cleansing. Use this colour if you have a tumour.*

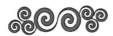

Turquoise - *immune strengthener. Cools fever and any inflammation.*

Blue - *insomnia, rest, and relaxation.*

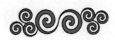

Violet - *beauty, dignity, and enhances self-esteem.*

Magenta - *to let go of negativity of any description.*

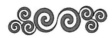

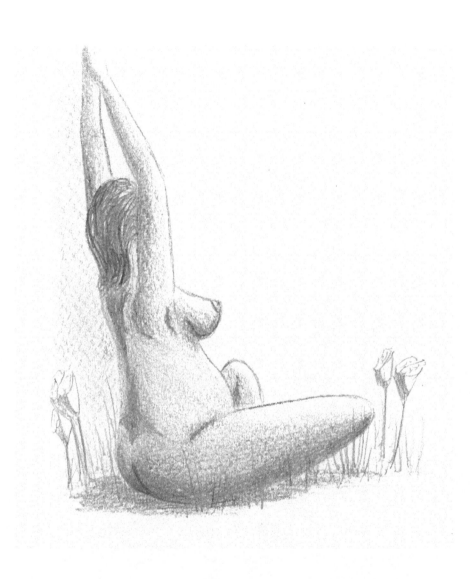

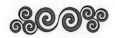

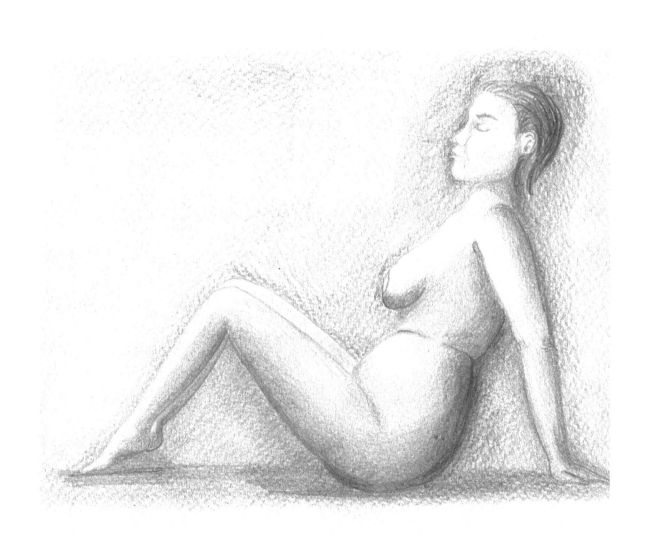

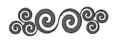

Moon Week

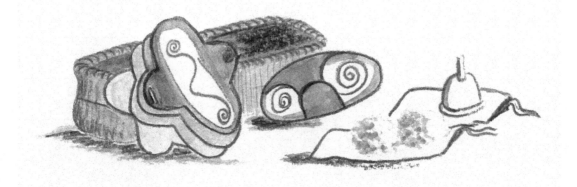

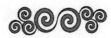

Day One

This is the first day of your Moon Week. Prepare to pamper yourself. This week you belong to no one but Grandmother Moon! Take the phone off the hook. Fill a bath, and add essential oil of geranium or jasmine or lavender.

Meanwhile, make a pot of chamomile or lavender tea. Play some Baroque music. Light a white candle to honour the Moon Goddess. Say some loving affirmations. Choose some from the list of power thoughts (which begin on page 103). Perhaps you can make your own cards to carry with you or even record some to listen to in the bath. This will allow you to access your deepest feelings and thoughts. Afterwards, pick up your journal and start writing about what it was like to nurture yourself in this way.

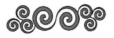

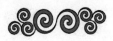

Day Two

Take a walk in Nature on your own. Find somewhere quiet to sit. Fill your heart with gratitude for the great Earth. Thank Mother Nature. Really feel this gratitude well up in your heart.

Close your eyes, and bless the Moon. Ask her to guide your body into its natural rhythm.

What does "rhythm" mean? Explore the word, and the feelings associated with it, including your own rhythm and that of the Earth, the Moon, the Universe. Say "rhythm" out loud. What energy does it send into the space around you?

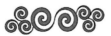

Connect to the Moon.
Accept and celebrate the blood. Shame no more. Connect with Nature, instinct and intuition.
Accept, instead of deny.
Hills, rivers, rain and sunshine.
Seasons: flow with them instead of trying to hide.
Connect with the life-death cycle.
We have lost touch
Allow the positive
Allow energy and power through
Cast off the shame attached to menstruation, and celebrate!

\- Helen, Cycle to the Moon workshop participant

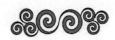

Day Three

What negative body images do you still hold? Write down all your negative beliefs, and then burn them! Do this privately, or invite friends to your Burning Bowl ceremony. Perhaps they too could release their thoughts which keep them tied to negative thinking? Afterwards, write a list of positive ideas and experiences you'd like to associate with menstruation.

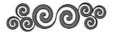

How do you look when you have your period? Do you wriggle into a tracksuit and hide beneath the covers? How would you like to look? If you work all day in an office, then maybe the best thing you can do is slide into bed in your tracksuit or pyjamas and nurture yourself. Be aware of how you treat yourself. Take as much pride in yourself as you might at any other time of the month. Think about beauty, nurture, self-care, hygiene and rest.

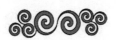

What can you do to make Moon week easier and more gentle for you? Put this into action. Write down at least five things.

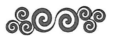

Day Four

If you don't bleed on day four, but continue again on day five, your adrenal glands are not functioning properly.

When you get out of bed first thing in the morning, stand naked in front of a full-length mirror. Say, "I love you. I love you. I love you." Even when your hair is messy, your mouth is dry, your tummy is bloated, and you feel groggy, make time to SMILE at yourself and say "Hey there, you! You're lookin' good, girlfriend!"

Draw yourself standing in front a mirror, naked.
(Try and have fun with your picture!)

YOU ARE DIVINELY BEAUTIFUL!!

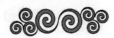

Devise a self-care schedule for this month. Learning to love includes nurturing ourselves with simple, unprocessed foods, and taking time to be alone for quiet contemplation. It means finding enjoyable and creative ways to exercise. Self-care is about saying 'yes' to yourself. It is about relaxing sleep, and pursuing leisure interests. Self-care is about following your dreams.

You know best what will nurture you and help you to thrive in this modern world. Schedule at least two nurturing activities for each day. Feel free to add more! Don't forget things like brushing your skin or stopping to smell the roses. Reminder notes about drinking plenty of spring water, and eating raw, fresh fruit and vegetables, could be part of your plan.

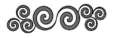

Day Five

Take yourself to dinner. Dress up. Light a candle, play some music ~ perhaps some lively salsa music ~ and eat the most delicious food that appeals to you. You deserve a treat. Dinner can and does taste fantastic on your own. Make it a priority to have time out, regardless of whether you are single, or married with ten children.

Create a list of 100 ideas which will help you feel great! And don't forget to do them. Even one a day will make all the difference.

(Here are four to start you off)

1. bellydancing
2. sleeping in on a rainy morning snuggled beneath the duvet
3. feeding the ducks at the park
4. remembering the simplicity of life by keeping a gratitude journal, and writing down five things each day that you're grateful for

_____

_____

_____

_____

_____

_____

_____

_____

_____

_____

_____

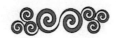

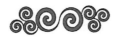

If you're still bleeding, make sure you indulge in a passion. Try doing one or two of the things listed in your 100 things that make you feel great! Don't forget warm baths, solitude, and nourishing music to fill your senses! Write down how you feel at the end of Moon week. What have you learnt about yourself? What might you do differently next month?

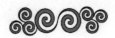

Retreats for Moon Week

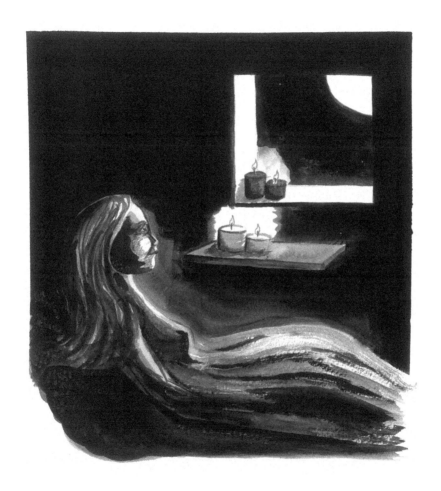

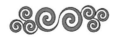

Snuggling up in Bed

Give yourself permission to crawl under the blankets. Afterwards, write down how this feels. Are you relaxed, bored, comforted, safe? Perhaps you feel guilt about being in bed during the daytime. In what ways can you make your bedroom a comfy nest? A healthy bedroom is one which has no electrical impulses or mobile phones. Leave your laptop, Kindle, smartphone and other devices well away from where you sleep.

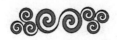

Long Candlelit Baths

Just you, some candles, perhaps gentle music, and a few drops of essential oil in a tub of lovely warm water. Dim the lights. Allow yourself to soak and unwind. Close your eyes, and let your body relax. Allow yourself to have an Epsom salts bath at least once a week. This is not only deeply nourishing, but will help boost your magnesium levels.

Later, write down what it's like to pamper yourself in this way. Did you have any revelations?

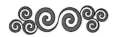

Walk in Solitude in Nature

Even if you can only spare ten minutes, find a way to rest in the arms of Mother Nature. Feel her under your bare feet, touch the bark of an ancient oak tree, let the sunshine warm your skin, and feel the wind on your face. Leave your cares behind, and be a child of Nature. Write down your experience of letting go and becoming one with the Ultimate Mother. Has she spoken to you? What did she say?

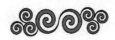

Meditation and Stillness

Meditation doesn't necessarily involve sitting, yogi-like, with legs crossed and chanting. Simply closing your eyes and allowing thoughts to dissipate will bring you to a place of calm. Let your breath slow down, and make each inhale and exhale conscious and deep. Write down how you feel after at least five minutes of bringing stillness to your mind and body. Did you feel comfortable being still? Did you want to do something else? How might five minutes of stillness each day change your life? Be mindful of excuses not to be still, and if you keep coming up with reasons to do something else, ask yourself: what am I running away from?

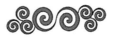

Psychic Energy

Learn to close your eyes, and simply listen. Being in Nature, taking a shower, or doing something creative, such as cooking, can open us to bursts of intuition and inspiration. Take notes! I often have my most intuitive moments when taking out the compost! Perhaps it's something to do with being barefoot on the grass, hearing the birdsong, and letting the wind whisper words into my ears.

Have you noticed when/where you're most in touch with your Higher Self?

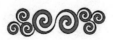

Going for a Moon walk

Allow yourself the pleasure of walking beneath the light of the Moon. Feel her, breathe her, stare at her in awe. How does it feel to connect with Grandmother Moon on this starry night? If this becomes a regular ritual, how might it change you?

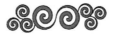

Adorning the Red Goddess

You are a goddess! Adorn yourself. You might wear red clothing or jewellery or lipstick, or perhaps you'd prefer to make a garland with flowers. How does it feel to pamper yourself?

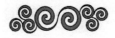

Wearing Red Underwear

Red is the colour of life. Treat yourself to some new underwear. What does it feel like to specifically wear red pants during your menstrual cycle? Go on girl, get your sassy pants on! Have fun, and allow the wild woman in you to come out and play.

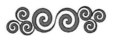

Red Thread

Regardless of where you are on the menstrual trinity, why not buy or make some red jewellery? It could be a ruby, garnet or beads made from red felt, glass or wood. How do you feel when wearing your 'colour of life' jewellery? Why did you choose these particular pieces?

In the Blessingway ceremonies I officiate, the women weave a red thread of hemp or wool. If you're part of a Red Tent group, or are having a menarche ceremony, you might like to weave a red thread.

Red is the colour of blood, and is what links all humans throughout time. During the red-thread ritual, pass the ball to the guest of honour. She wraps it around her wrist several times, and then throws the ball across the circle to one of her guests. That woman also wraps it around her wrist several times before throwing it to someone else in the circle. This continues until everyone is linked into the web. Aftewards, the celebrant then cuts the thread between each person.

By wrapping the string around your wrist several times, you'll have enough to be able to make a braid/plait from it so that it sits more comfortably around the wrist later on. I like how the braid becomes 'felted' after being worn for a few weeks, and I have quite a few which are now used as bookmarks. You can use this bracelet each Moon week.

The red thread reminds us of the story of Tantrika, the Spider Goddess, and how she weaved the world. As we weave our circle of sisterhood, we come together all through the One Mother. If you've had a red-thread ceremony as part of a Red Tent group, then even after the string is cut, you'll remember that we all still come from the same ball of yarn.

In Native American myth, The Spider Grandmother (Spider Woman), created all life by spinning her web, and connected all living life together using her magical thread.

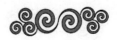

Red Food

This is such a fun way to really get a sense of red from the earth. Write down a list of all the red fruits and vegetables that you have access to, and describe how you feel when eating them.

Lighting a Red Candle on your Menstrual Altar

Maiden, you might like to light a white candle and a red candle.

Crone, you might like to light a white, red and black candle to represent the menstrual trinity.

Give yourself time and space to be with your altar. Allow the light to fill you with a sense of the sacred. Describe your experience.

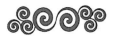

Sex during the Moontime

For so long, and in so many ways, there have been countless taboos around menstruation, not least of which is having sex while you're bleeding. Some cultures, such as the Hopi, Omaha, and Navajo, also believe that you're more likely to conceive during menstruation.

Many women have found that making love during their Moon Week is deeply relaxing and eases their cramps. If you can let go of cultural taboos around this, then you might just find yourself feeling more liberated as you open your legs and bleeding yoni to your lover. It's a pretty rare man that would decline sex just because of a bit of blood. The Yin Juice of your body will nourish him.

"Roll out the red carpet"
comes from the ancient woman-craft
of consecrating ceremonies
with menstrual blood.

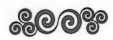

The Menstrual Mind

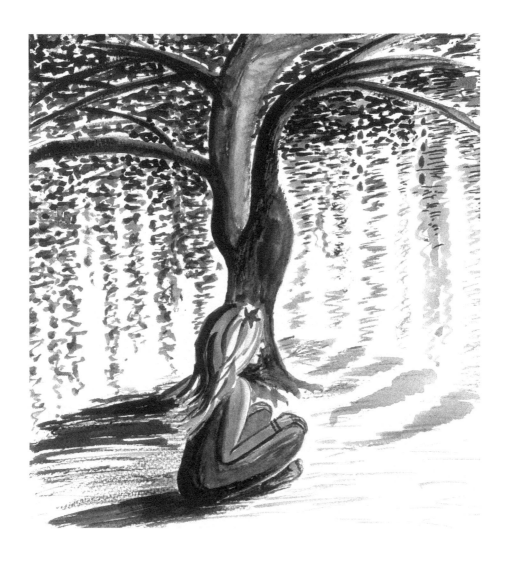

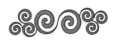

"Isolate yourself during the flow. It is your time to acquire spiritual energy."

~ Old Menstrual Law.

Menstruation deeply links the body, mind and soul. Don't forget the importance of 'bodymind' in all your work to release menstrual taboos. Pick one of the following 'power thoughts' for each month from the following pages. Focus on what it means for you. Write down your immediate response, positive or negative. Spend a couple of minutes free-writing without lifting your pen from the page. Afterwards, decide how you might incorporate it into your life and into your Moon cycle.

Use the blank pages to stick pictures, drawings and photos, and write out the affirmation to support your new thinking.

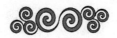

I am a strong and powerful woman.

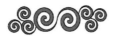

I love my body and my body loves me!

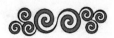

My body now bleeds in time with the Moon.

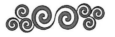

Bleeding is natural.

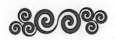

My body is pure and holy.

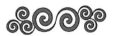

My period is easy and gentle.

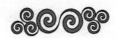

I relax and let my body fall into the Moon's cycle.

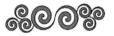

I am deeply linked to Grandmother Moon
regardless of where I am on the menstrual trinity.

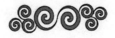

I gracefully accept the cyclical nature of my body.

If you have been through many of the exercises in this book and are still hanging onto someone else's attitudes, try doing the following healing ritual.

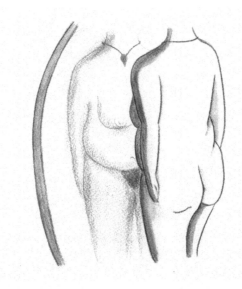

It works just as well individually in front of a mirror, or by sharing it with a close friend or in a women's circle, such as a Red Tent. If sharing with others, begin by sitting down and making eye contact. Hold hands, and remember to breathe, breathe, breathe, deeply. Lift the words from the page. Feel them. Keep eye contact. When you're ready, move to the front of the mirror and look into your eyes. Remember to keep breathing deeply. Witnessing each other's mirror work is amazingly powerful and healing. Bring tissues!

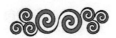

I Am a Beautiful Woman
A Healing Ceremony

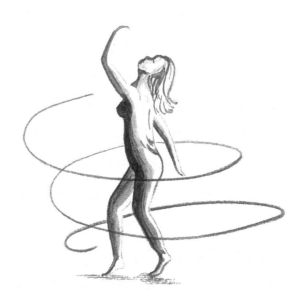

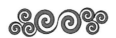

If you feel drawn to it, you can begin the ceremony by following an olden-day gypsy ritual: rubbing lemon peels on your heels and ankles. It is believed to bring purification.

Today I give myself permission to heal. I allow myself to truly see who I am.
I am proud to be a woman and female.
[Are you breathing deeply?]

I am a child of the Goddess. I am remembering my Goddess nature.
[Breathe.]

Today I allow myself the freedom to honour the sanctity of my beautiful body.
I celebrate and honour my womanhood.
[Remember to breathe!]

The shame of my foremothers does not belong to me.
I am no longer ashamed of any part of myself.
[Breathe.]

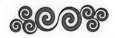

I am a woman now. Today I hold my inner girl inside my heart where I can protect her.
I know she is always safe, perfect and whole.
[Take a long deep breath.]

I am wise. I am worthy.
I am remembering that I am a wild woman!
[Is your breathing deep and slow?]

On this day, I choose to forgive my mother for her misunderstanding of menstruation.
I forgive my grandmothers for their misunderstanding of menstruation.
And I forgive their mothers.
I forgive myself.
Instead, I choose to remember my ancestresses
who understood the beauty of being female.
[How is your breathing?]

With an open heart, I honour and embrace my femininity.
At my deepest cellular memory,
where I know what it means to be a woman, I love myself.
[Breathe.]

I choose to create my own beliefs about menstruation.
I am remembering that I am free.
[Keep breathing.]

I am a beautiful woman.
[Long, slow, deep breaths.]

I honour myself for the courage
it has taken to get to this part of my life.
[Breathe.]

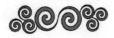

I no longer give others permission to oppress me.
Today I forgive, and I am free.
[Breathe.]

I am beautiful. I am a woman.
I am a goddess. I am wild. I am free.
Today and every day.
[Breathe.]

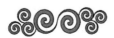

Chakra Meditation

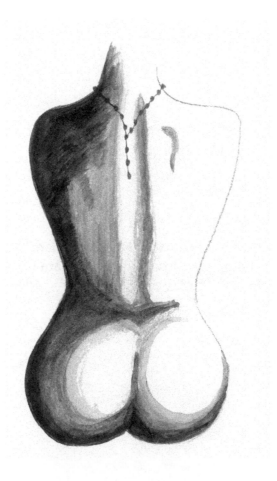

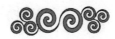

The word chakra comes from the ancient Sanskrit language. Eight chakra (chakrum is singular, chakra is plural) exist in alignment along the spine. They essentially collect the light from our aura. Just as the aura that surrounds us maintains our life energy, so too do the chakra. The colours of the aura funnel into each chakrum.

* Familiarise yourself with each one, in terms of colour, position and qualities.

Imagine a small plate or disc of luminous, pure colour. As you do this, imagine each chakrum opening up like a flower opens from a tight bud. Explore the colour and breathe it into your body. Do this slowly and deeply. This is a colour-breathing technique. Close the flower into a bud before moving onto the next one, or close them from top to bottom when you've been through them all.

Start with the base.

Base chakrum - *Red* - known as the sexuality chakrum, it relates to creativity, passion and life force.
Sacral - *Orange* - our genes are reflected in the activity and energy of this 'earthly' chakrum, as is our wellness and happiness.
Solar plexus - *Yellow* - represents sensitivity. If we have unresolved situations, we will feel it here 'in our gut'. Our self-esteem level is seated here.
Heart - *Green* - harmony and love. Our real self shines through here. Green gives us a sense of balance.
Thymus - *Turquoise* brings generosity and life.
Throat (thyroid) - *Blue* is an expression of sound, truth and communication.
Brow (pituitary) - *Violet* helps transmits the energy of the pituitary gland. It is here you are able to receive your intuition from your Higher Self. Known as the Third Eye.
Crown (pineal) - *Magenta* - Here we find the perfection chakrum. It is the centre of our spirituality, and our connection to the Divine.

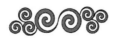

In a lot of languages,

the words God, menstruation, blood,

sacred and Moon are the same word!

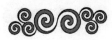

The Menstrual Muse

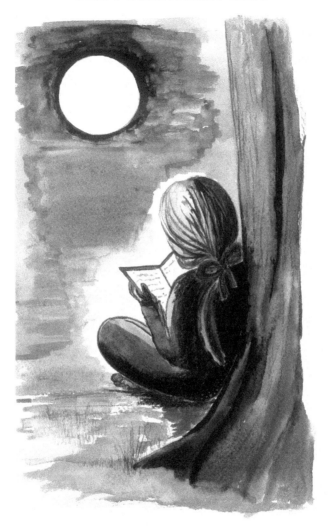

Every country, every religion, has women and Moon-linked symbolism and imagery.

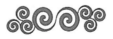

Allow yourself ten to fifteen minutes to walk quietly around your home, garden or community. Find three items which are symbolic of the positve way in which your see your cycle, and one item that is negative, whether for you personally, or as our culture sees it. Bring them back home and make these symbols into a story, either written or verbal, to share with a friend or write in your journal. For example, a rag doll because it reminds you of wanting to snuggle up in bed and be a little girl again: mother's love and nurturing. A dirty sock may remind you of all the negativity you've been led to believe about menstruation: filthy, unhygienic.

1.)
2.)
3.)
4.)

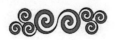

Write your story... and then use the blank pages which follow to record your ebb and flow.

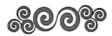

Moontime Moontime
Hometime
my body is ripe and full
I can feel the first stirrings inside me
sense a spirit coming closer
I am afraid...fear - white clinical rooms
nameless faces
empty spaces, empty spaces
no one to hold my hand. All those years I tried to hide this womanliness
to hide my new ripening, as my mother said goodbye to hers.
This blood made me an enemy so became my enemy.
Now it is time to prepare my body for real, spiritual children
and to finally enter womanhood.
I am afraid I will not be able to love, to nurture
"Oh, my child," she whispers to me...
"You are not alone, I am with you.
Light a candle for me, sing to the Moon
Take my hand and laugh, love.
Tears fall from grief, release, loss, Love."

- Vikki, Cycle to the Moon workshop participant

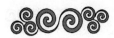

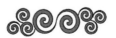

My body is pure and holy. My body does not contain my soul. It is my soul.
So when a man makes love to me, he meets my woman soul.
My body is beautiful.
My body is female; it holds deep, dark secret places; deep, dark caves and hollows.

Sally, Cycle to the Moon workshop participant

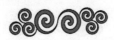

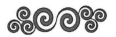

I like the way my husband has always been comfortable with my menstruation...
maybe because I was comfortable with it myself, so it was no big deal.
I don't know how he learned about it.
It is such a big secret in some families...even for women.
When our daughter Karen got her first period,
he was the first to know after me.
I'm not sure how he felt, seeing his daughter as a sexual being.
We lit a red candle at the dinner table and each had a glass of wine to celebrate!

Gill, Cycle to the Moon workshop participant

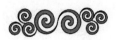

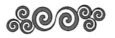

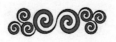

The Visitor by Veronika Sophia Robinson

In velvet gown of deep, blood red
I come again, riding high upon crimson tide, soft and silent in the night
Whispering my return.
A long absence it's been...
Did you think the flow of milk from your swollen, stretch-marked breasts
could keep me away forever?
I'm back!
Time to hold hands with your sisters and cycle to the Moon.
I spiral down, slow and sweet, into black moss
Unaware of my return, dampness, you think, from lover's early morning touch
I stain your fingers slippery pink.
"Oh, you're back" you moan gently into the morning light, when you realise I'm there.
You fear my return. I'm ripening your womb for a fertility feast!
Don't you remember how we played?
Like the grand finale curtain call, I announce the end of every scene.
Onto the stage they dance: an ovarian princess
no rehearsal, enter a cast of thousands; each a willing escort.
Russian roulette. Hit and miss.
You await an explosion...time ticking.
And then I waltz along in velvet gown of deep, blood red
Riding upon a crimson tide, I come again....
Your friend!

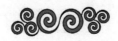

On the eve of your period take time to hear the muse. Allow the poet in you to step out of the cupboard. Try writing at different times in your menstrual cycle. Our creative expression ebbs and flows and expresses rather differently at various stages of our cycle. After menopause, we may become more conscious of the Moon's cycle weaving through our daily life if we haven't already done so.

Ninety percent of Western women suffer some form of menstrual discomfort, ranging from slight to severe. Allopathic medicine can offer no explanation for this, and offers no cure. To be clear, the pills, drugs and hormones offered by doctors will not cure you. They act as a band-aid. Only a change of lifestyle and attitude will bring you relief from menstrual discomfort each month.

Try eating seasonal food for a few months, and feel the difference both in terms of your conscious awareness of the Earth's cycles, but also in how your body feels when eating local food. Write down what changes you notice. Have you remedied nutritional deficiencies by incorporating more mineral and vitamin-rich foods, beverages and supplements into your diet?

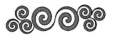

Write down a list of the foods which are available abundantly in your local area for each season of the year. Can you supplement shop-bought produce by growing some of your own foods?

Spring

Summer

Autumn

Winter

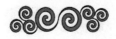

Modern statistics relating to menstruating woman
are taken from huge cities
about women whose lifestyles
are not in accord with Nature.

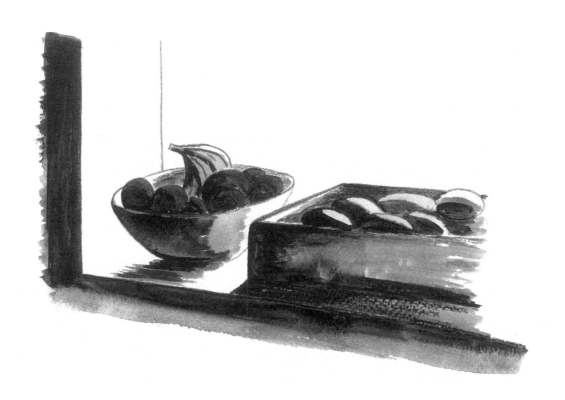

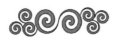

Keeping a journal is an effective way of looking at the fabric of your life: the highs, the lows, and the in betweens. This sacred space is not for judgement. It is, quite simply, a place to pause for reflection: a place to learn from. If you want more space than this book, something as simple as a spiral notebook for daily writing can change your whole outlook on life. Maybe you could make it a theme journal? Perhaps you will study the seasons and observe them with all your senses? A 'feelings' journal will help you understand your emotions. A gratitude journal where you write down at least five things each day to be thankful for is incredibly life affirming. How about a nutrition journal? The more you study natural foods, the more you'll be amazed that the human body has everything it needs for healing right outside your front door.

I wear a red dress to deny my shame
I am a woman and I am proud, strong, creative
Harness this power
like riding the white horses of the ocean
To sing in starlight
I create naturally

Vikki, Cycle to the Moon workshop participant

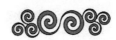

Rituals for Modern Women

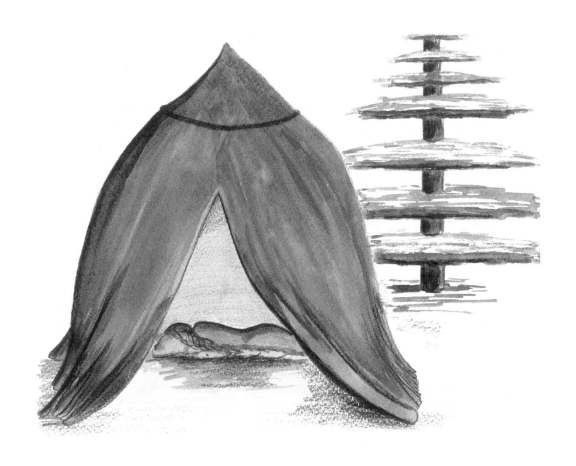

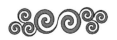

Rituals for Modern Women

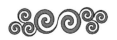

The human spirit loves and needs ritual. It can be something as simple as lighting a candle or as elaborate as a communal celebration. The rituals included here can be adapted and personalised to suit your individual or group's needs. Write or improvise your ceremony.

Full Moon Prayer for the Red Tent

Goddess of the White Moon, shine down on me. Shine down on all my sisters.

Join us together, and let our great bleeding be in honour of you and of ourselves.

Show us how to self-love and self-care. Join with us as we say this prayer.

After invoking the Moon Goddess, gather in a circle to form the shape of a full Moon. Bring a gift to symbolise the power of women. You might also like to gift the circle with a white flower, and to wear white clothing.

Each woman takes a turn to light a white candle and places in it front of her. Gather fresh herbs of lavender, rosemary and mint, and place them in a basin with spring water. Wash each other's feet, and brush hair as a symbol of nurturing. Sing or chant and share your dreams.

A New Moon Ritual

Invoke your own Higher Self as you do this ceremony, either on your own or within a small circle. Obtain some apple wood and carve your initials into the bark. Place the wood under your pillow, and sleep with it for three nights before the new Moon. Carry it with you by day. If there is a deep wish or desire, ordain it with the wood.

On the eve of the new Moon, go to an area of water, such as a small pond or lake, for example, and cast the wood into the water. This dream wood is now free to return to the earth with your vibration. Finish the ritual with a short prayer of gratitude.

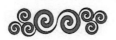

Moon Flow Ritual

You can choose to collect some or all of your Moon blood in containers for releasing onto the earth. Perhaps you can create a garden specifically dedicated to honouring the woman in you. Red roses or some other blood-red flower would be a visual reminder of the blood given to our Earth Mother. Invite the plant deva to nurture this piece of dedicated land. Alternatively, you can make your plot of land in something as simple as a pot plant or the base of a tall tree.

Burning Bowl Ritual

The phoenix ceremony (burning bowl) is a time of letting go and renewal. Write a list of everything in your life you wish to release: debt, toxic relationships, poor health, painful periods, cramps, headaches, and so on. Burn this paper in a fireproof bowl or a firepit in the garden. Create your own chant. Play some music. Feel the relief of letting go. Tomorrow, write a list of what you want to create in your life to replace the negativity.

Light of the Moon

To stimulate ovulation, use the light of the full Moon, or indirect lighting such as candles, or a low lamp, in your bedroom, at days 14, 15 and 16 of your cycle. (Ensure the candles are in a safe, fireproof container.)

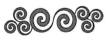

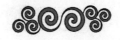

Moon Dreamer

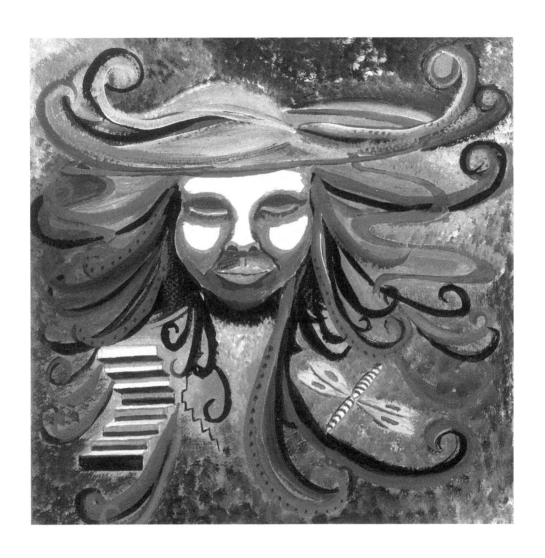

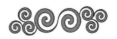

Moontime opens up our intuition.

By allowing ourselves to honour this time,

we can eliminate premenstrual tendencies.

In many tribal villages, Moontime is a sacred passage leading

to a greater awareness of self.

When we cycle to the Moon, we menstruate approximately every 29.5 days. That there is so much variation on this in the Western world is a strong indicator of the impact of modern living and the stresses we endure. Use the length of your cycle as an indicator of where your body is at (but please don't beat yourself up if it is longer or shorter).

When we are in tune with our body and cycle, we can feel ourselves ovulating. There is such a wide variance in cycle length these days that doctors consider it normal to bleed any time. *It might be normal but it is not natural.* Modern statistics relating to menstruating woman are taken from huge cities about women whose lifestyles are not in accord with Nature. Artificial street lighting, pollution, stress, foods coated in chemicals, nutritional deficiencies, are just a few contributing factors in the variance of cycle days.

Our body's cycle is regulated by the Moon's light. The pituitary and hypothalamus glands are light sensitive, which is why we disrupt our cycle immensely by sleeping near artificial light, such as street lights, computer, mobile/cell phone or clock-radio lights. In fact, keep all electromagnetic devices well out of your sleeping space. If you intend to be conscious of cycling to the Moon, and ensuring optimal health, then don't sleep under or next to any artificial light. Instead, keep your room dark, and only open your curtain for the week of the full Moon, thus coming into alignment with it. If you live in the country it will not be necessary to keep out starlight. Just to reiterate, city girls often begin menstruation earlier than country girls because of street lighting.

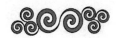

Describe your sleeping arrangements. Is there room for improvement, such as allowing in natural light? What are you drinking in the evening? Does alcohol or caffeine/chocolate or tannin (tea) play a regular role in your dietary intake?

Take notes, and over the course of a few months you'll see a pattern emerge. This provides you with the raw ingredients to make changes to create optimal health at all levels of your being.

We suffer

when we hide

menstruation.

Let your bleeding time speak to you. Listen. Understanding the Moon's cycles will give you an idea of how your own moods, emotions, sensations, dreams and thoughts change over the course of a menstrual month.

New Moon: seeds, ideas, hopes, beginning projects.

Quarter Moon: manifesting the ideas and projects which were conceived at the New Moon.

Full Moon: a time for completing; giving birth to the New Moon's intentions.

Three-quarter Moon: provides us with understanding of the many manifestations we've created.

Dark Moon: letting go, transformation.

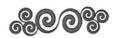

Dreaming

If you don't remember your dreams when you wake up each morning, it is a sign that you're low on vitamin B6. A deficiency in this vitamin will also manifest in menstrual disturbances.

Pre-ovulation Dreams:

_____

_____

_____

_____

_____

_____

_____

_____

_____

_____

_____

_____

_____

_____

_____

_____

_____

_____

_____

_____

_____

_____

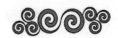

Ovulation Dreams:

_____
_____
_____
_____
_____
_____
_____
_____
_____
_____
_____
_____
_____
_____
_____
_____
_____
_____
_____
_____
_____
_____
_____
_____
_____
_____
_____
_____

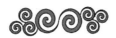

Premenstruation Dreams:

_____
_____
_____
_____
_____
_____
_____
_____
_____
_____
_____
_____
_____
_____
_____
_____
_____
_____
_____
_____
_____
_____
_____

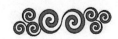

Menstruation Dreams:

_____
_____
_____
_____
_____
_____
_____
_____
_____
_____
_____
_____
_____
_____
_____
_____
_____
_____
_____
_____
_____
_____
_____
_____
_____
_____

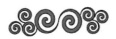

In the UK, most menstruating women
use between 286 and 358 pads
or tampons per year.

Ninety-eight percent of these
are flushed down the toilet,
and end up polluting the environment.

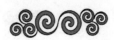

Catching Our Blood

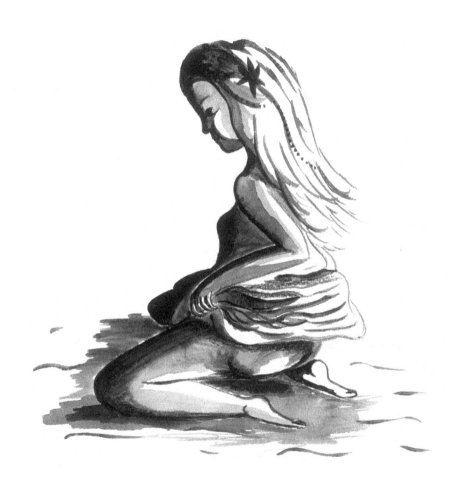

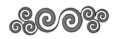

Many of us have been indoctrinated with menstruation as something which must be hidden away and not talked about. Advertisements for our bodily cycles teach us that menstruation is a medical condition for which we must use bleach-white tampons and pads; and, sadly, that ovulation's cervical mucus should be caught in fragrant mini-pads. Cubicles in public toilets have special containers to destroy our 'hazardous' waste. All aspects of our cycle are integral to our sexuality. Why are we hiding any part of it away? What are we telling ourselves each time we use a disposable pad or tampon? Bleeding is intrinsic to being a sexually mature woman. If we take a holistic approach to this, then we'll see beautiful ways in which we can connect with Mother Earth, such as consciously catching our blood.

A tampon 'plugs' us up at a time when we're designed to let our bodily blood seep away from us. Women who move over to cloth pads or a Moon cup (which catches blood, and doesn't absorb the vaginal secretions) find their cycle becoming easier. They're more in touch with themselves. My friend, the late Jeannine Parvati Baker, wrote beautifully of menstruation when she said: *The pad becomes a canvas onto which you pour the paint of your being.* Beautiful! Our yoni makes art!

In short, when we hold the flow back, we're opening ourselves up to all sort of diseases. We are more than just the physical body, but are emotional, psychological and spiritual beings, too. This is why we need to be mindful of all the ways we distance ourselves from our blood. We need to *see* our blood, to *touch* it, and to be able to *smell* it in order to access the limbic part of our brain. Germaine Greer once suggested *tasting* your blood, if you consider yourself a sexually liberated feminist. Your Moontime can be as deeply rewarding as any other aspect of your sexuality. The choice is yours, but that will only happen if you liberate yourself from menstrual taboos and other people's fears and disgust about menstruation.

One of the things I most enjoy about bleeding onto a cloth pad is that after they've soaked in a bucket for a couple of hours, I pour the soak water/blood onto my houseplants, or herbs in the garden. My fruit trees rather like it, too. It's nutrient rich, and a wonderful natural fertiliser. And, it's free!

Yoni Art

Just as blood on our pad is art, we can also make yoni art onto paper.

Yoni is a Sanskrit word, which means vagina or womb. It is considered a divine passage or sacred temple. Use natural earth paints or even better, your own menstrual blood, to take a print of the entrance to your yoni. Let those lovely lips kiss the paper! Use beautiful parchment paper and make as many prints as you like. Don't be shy! This is the ultimate in self-love. Feel free to frame it and hang it up on a wall, or use it as a bookmark. Be proud of your gorgeous body. Every square inch of it! We can only change cultural taboos one beautiful yoni at a time. Let's start here.

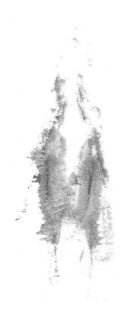

Put a copy of your yoni art here as a keepsake.

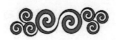

In the UK, most menstruating women use between 286 and 358 pads or tampons per year. Ninety-eight percent of these are flushed down the toilet, and end up polluting the environment. Fifty-two percent of these are released, untreated, into the sea. Tampons require six months to biodegrade. Pads take longer. The plastic liners on sanitary pads don't break down.

Since the dawn of humanity, women have been creatively catching their menstrual blood. Somewhere along the way we have been convinced that our blood is something to be hidden away, and something to be despised. With the advent of the multi-billion pound disposable menstrual products industry came a host of ailments and diseases associated with the toxins (and cultural shame of our cycle), not to mention a devastating impact on the environment. This is something which affects us all. Our genital area is sensitive, and exposure to chemicals can lead to discomfort and major health issues. Limiting contact with dioxin and other toxins is in every woman's best interests. Even low levels of toxins have been implicated with things such as endometriosis, immune disorders, cancer, pelvic-inflammatory disease, hormone changes, and reduced fertility. Caring about your body and caring about the Earth that your granddaughters will inherit are steps toward making choices which take you away from disposable menstrual products. The cloth pad is back! Made of soft, natural fabrics in appealing colours and patterns, you can use organic fabrics or ones from traditional agriculture which don't use chemicals, pesticides and insecticides.

Cloth pads can last for a decade or longer (I have some which are fifteen years old!), depending on the care, and the type of fabric used. Most women would go through seven to 12 pads during a cycle. Sew yourself a collection of eco-friendly, pretty pads in soft, brushed cotton, hemp or bamboo in patterns of your choice: floral, tartan, stripes, teddy bears. I even have one with Santa Claus! Gives a whole new meaning to the Gentleman in Red coming down the chimney! Women who use cloth pads regularly report that their periods become lighter. This sewing pattern uses an optional nylon lining to improve the leak-proofness of the pad. It can be reused in the future, at the end of the lifespan of the fabric. Use tracing paper to go over the pattern.

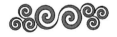

Sew your own reuseable cloth menstrual pads

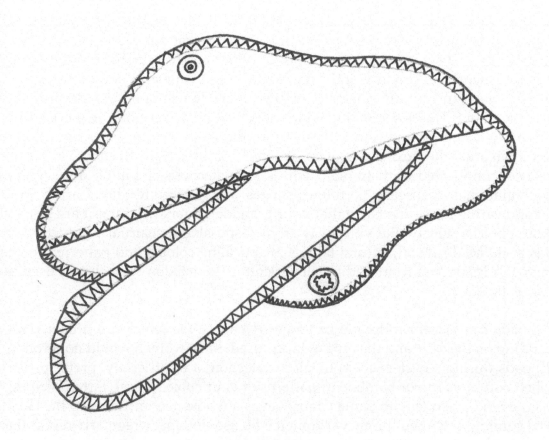

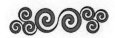

Care

Cloth pads are easy to care for. Simply soak for a couple of hours in a bucket, then rinse by hand before including them in your normal wash with other clothes. The soak water is a great nutrient for your houseplants, or garden plants. You might be squeamish at first, if you've only ever used tampons or disposable pads, but you'll get used to it. Even the resident male in our home has been known to handwash my cloth pads. Ah, true love.

If it helps you to put cloth pads into perspective, remember this: women in Third World countries who don't have access to pads, use sand or ash to catch their blood. If you'd like to help more women around the world use cloth pads, see our resource section for the *Not Just a Cloth Pad* project.

How to use

Unlike disposable pads, cloth pads are extremely absorbent and don't create a horrible odour. Therefore, you can leave them in place all day, or replace once if you've got a heavier flow. Use a fresh pad at night.

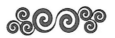

Method:

1.   Cut three of piece A from cotton fabric, and another one from nylon.

2.   Trim one piece to become piece B, and one piece to become piece C. Piece C is the opposite to piece B, so that together they make the top, with the envelope opening, through which you insert the inner absorbent pad.

3.   Neaten the long edges of B and C, so that they won't fray (machine zigzag or single-turn hem).

4.   Assemble the pad, and pin together in the following order:

•   piece A nylon, underneath

•   piece A cotton, right side of fabric uppermost

•   piece B, right-side down, long edge folded over two centimetres

•   piece C, right-side down

5.   Stitch round outer edge of pad on seam line.

6.   Trim seam allowance, and turn right-side out through B/C opening.

7.   Topstitch through all the layers.

8.   Attach press stud fasteners to the wings.

9.   Cut inner pad of brushed cotton.

10.   Neaten around the edges to prevent fraying. Insert through opening (as seen in picture 1). The inner pad can be made thicker, and the pad itself can be made longer and wider, for heavier flow or post-partum use.

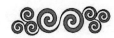

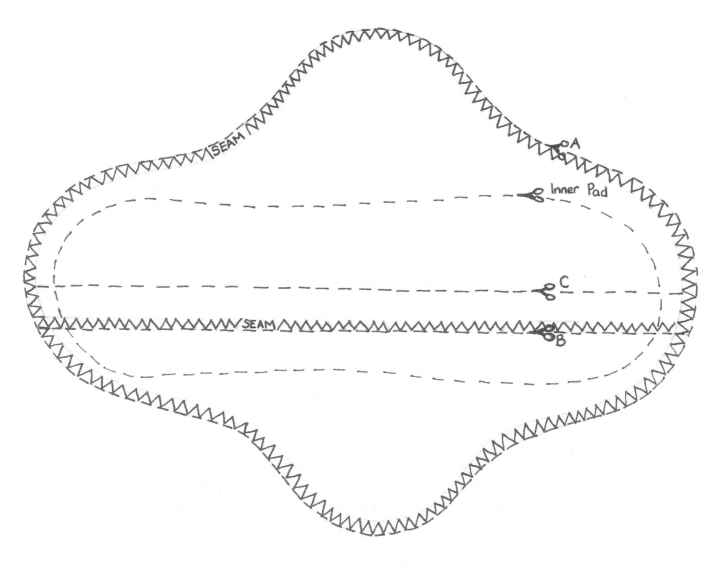

SEAM

A

Inner Pad

C

SEAM

B

Adjust the size to suit. Smaller for menarche; larger for post-partum bleeding.

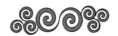

Finding our Way Home

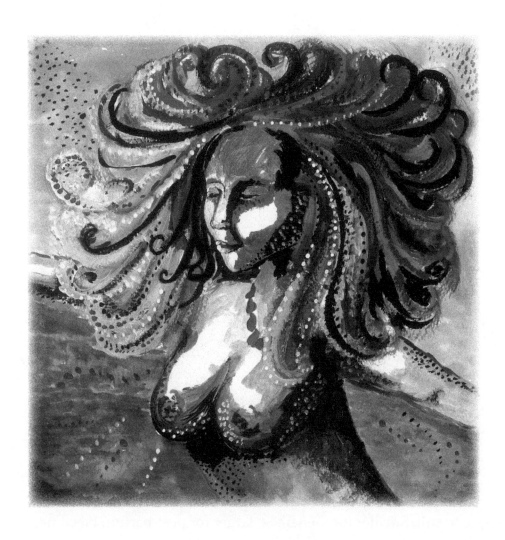

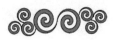

Connecting with Mother Earth

Earth provides us with a beautiful example of cyclical energy. Every year her canvas changes with the richness of the seasons: The beginning. The manifestation. The letting go, and the making way for the next phase. One of the many benefits of our modern culture is the availability of foods from around the world at any time of the year. On the surface, this seems like a wonderful thing. Dig a little deeper and we see many consequences of this, one example being a denial of what the body needs at certain times of the year.

Is it best for our bodies and the environment to eat strawberries in the middle of Winter? Or porridge on a mid-Summer's day?

Most of us do this all the time. And yet, if we were to eat seasonal foods our bodies would respond in kind. We'd make the connection with produce availability. By spending time in Nature, much more than many of us currently do, we'd tune in to our innate sense of Winter, Spring, Summer and Autumn. And we, too, would be familiar with lunar phases. It's no surprise that we're often unfamiliar with our body cycles when we're so out of touch with the natural cycles around us.

I trust my intuition and eat foods which support me.

I lovingly nurture my body.

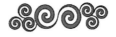

A treasure map or vision board depicts where you want to go or what you'd like to have. It's a collection of pictures and words or symbols, usually on card. A map can be as small as a business card or as large as your bedroom wall. Make the background colour appealing, and use bright pictures as opposed to black and white.

Create a map of how you'd like to experience Moon week, including body, mind and soul. You might include a picture of the full Moon with an affirmation: *I now bleed in harmony with Grandmother Moon. I choose to take this week to nurture myself and retreat with good books/ good company.*

You might include photos of yourself in a bathtub, or walking in Nature. Whatever images you use, make them positive and nurturing.

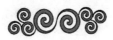

The Wise Crone

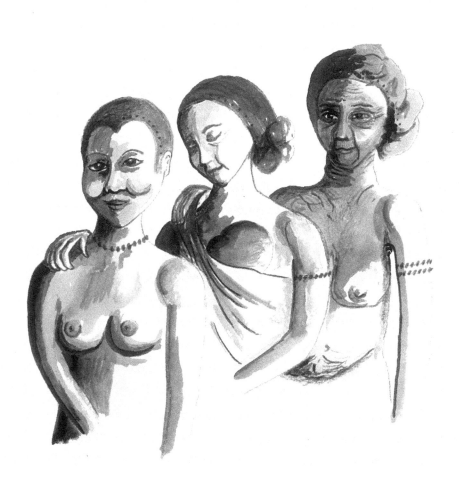

The Menstrual Trinity: maiden (loved), mother (lover), crone (beloved).

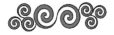

Menopause is a word that seems to strike fear into many Western women. It's associated with hot flushes, mood changes, sweats, nervousness, depression, low libido, and loss of self-esteem. Many women fear that they'll no longer be attractive, or not seen as sexually available. Does it have to be this way? Is this what Nature planned for women at the end of their reproductive lives? I don't believe so.

As our body eases up on producing the hormones associated with reproduction, the adrenal glands become the 'power' source of the body. If we were living naturally, we'd seamlessly glide from one phase of our menstrual life to the next. However, we live in a very stressful culture, and our adrenals work overtime: hence the symptoms often associated with 'the change'.

The main nutritional supplements for the flagging adrenals include Siberian ginseng, liquorice (not the candy), chromium, B-complex vitamins, vitamin C and magnesium. Try transdermal magnesium (you spray it on your skin, and it allows your body to absorb eight times the amount of magnesium than through foods). Eat calcium-rich food such as tahini, almonds, cabbage, sesame seed, broccoli, Brussels sprouts, and so on. Dairy is not, contrary to mainstream opinion, a good source of calcium. Beware of acid-forming foods such as alcohol, sugar, table salt (Celtic sea salt, for example, is fine), caffeine, chocolate, junk food; and smoking. Exercise each day. Try the Australian Bush Flower Essence *Macrocarpa*. It is very helfpul for the adrenals. Most importantly, let your creative self shine.

While menstruation is a personal journey, walking the path of the Crone is more planetary in energy. In her, we find the wise elder. The inner terrain of our journey to her may be invisible to others, but if we have engaged in self-care and fiercely stood by ourselves and honoured the sacred feminine, then we will experience first-hand that menopause is not an illness. It only becomes so if we have ignored the body's calls, our innate femininity, and dedication to well-being. What we haven't learnt in the menstrual years, we will be called to confront at menopause. The wild woman within comes to see that this is not a time to be domesticated and controlled, but to break free of bondage, personal and cultural.

How we prepare ourselves for menopause in the preceding years is as vital as the moment we step across the threshold to the Crone.

If ever there was a time for honesty in all areas of our lives, it is here. Instead of hot flushes, we will be blessed with an extraordinary level of creativity. Oh yes, we'll have power surges, but unlike anything our culture has warned us about!

Hot flushes and other menopausal 'symptoms' are not inevitable. They are warning signs: the consequences of ignoring bodily needs. If you've practised nutritional integrity, and your adrenals and thyroid are in a state of equilibrium, your surges will be of energy and creativity rather than that of the adrenals becoming stressed. Fundamental to physical ease during menopause is awareness, and making nurturing and self-care a priority during the menstrual years. Perimenopause is a gentle signal to check we're ready for the next big step in our lives.

At the gateway to the Crone we must acknowledge that the past is gone. We step into the new world. Surrender. Letting go. We may feel alone, but we are not. The Dark Goddess is waiting for us. Waiting for you. She has waited patiently to guide you.

Yes, do grieve for your old self if that's what you need to do. Grieve for babies never born from your body. Who you are now, right here, is the authentic you. Honour this journey with regular doses of therapeutic isolation. There is a reason why the journey is a solitary one. It's necessary for tapping into the unlimited energy which awaits. This is where we find our power. Here, in the wise years. The Crone recognises that her body is holy.

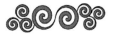

These yoga asanas can stimulate the adrenal glands:

Half Shoulder
Shoulder Stand
Child Pose
Hare Pose
Little Bird
Dog Pose
Abdominal Contractions
Dynamic Breath
Cobra/Sphinx
Bow
Fish
Bridge
Camel

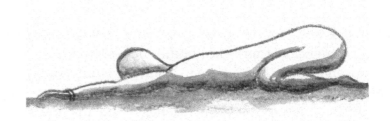

Menopause is a time for celebration; a time for new beginnings. We are (I hope) becoming wiser now. We're generally coming to the end of full-time mothering as our children leave the nest. We see the world differently. Yes, it may seem like an unknown world, but what a beautiful one! Here, we can take everything we've learned and experienced, and add our passion and freedom to the opportunities before us. Nature ordained that it would be a time of blessed spiritual growth: *a rebirth.*

We no longer bleed. Our wisdom is held within the body, and nourishes us. This is a gift. It is a journey into a sacred realm. There is no place or need for Hormone Replacement Therapy in the life of a consciously menopausal woman. Being called by the Crone is not a medical condition nor is it an illness. It is a key to freedom: the threshold to one of the most exciting times of your life. Any uncomfortable symptoms you experience are messages from the body asking you to pay attention, just like during menstruation. The same ideas apply nutritionally, but with a bigger emphasis on adrenal health.

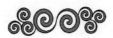

We talk of the Crone at menopause, but in many ways the years from 50 to 70 belong to *Maga*, and 70 onwards are the Crone years. The Maiden is represented by the archetype of Spring and the first-quarter Moon; the Mother resonates to the energy of Summer and the Full Moon; Maga to Autumn and the waning three-quarter Moon. The Crone finds her heart in the Dark Moon, Winter, and Solstice. She has seen the seasons, and lived through the turn of the Moon.

When is the best time to hold a ceremony to honour your Crone? For some women, they do so at age 50 or at 51, during their Chiron return. Chiron is known mythically as the Wounded Healer. Others do so a year after their periods have ceased. As an astrologer, I see the age of 56 as significant, when we experience our second Saturn return. You will know the right time for you.

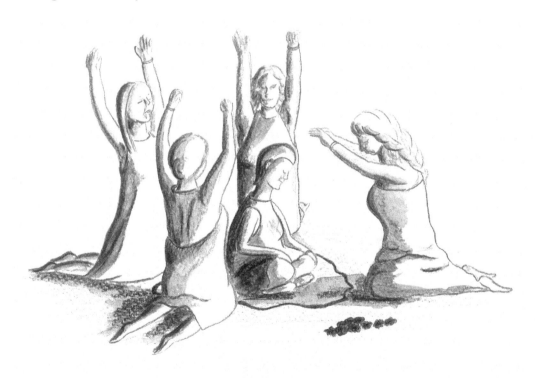

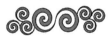

The Wise Crone Ceremony

In our culture, we're slowly starting to wake up and recognise that the Crone isn't some woman who is past her expiry date. No, not at all. She's sexy! She's wise! She's confident! She's smart! And we're going to honour her.

Our ancestresses knew her as the healer, the teacher, the leader. She was the Empowered One. Unlike your first Moonflow, or the birth of a baby, the Crone whispers her way into your life. She doesn't wave a flag saying 'This is your last period!' In many ways, it's a bit like child-led weaning. One day you realise it's been a while since your child last breastfed. 'Oh,' you softly say in recognition of the end of an era.

When we've walked hand in hand with our menstrual cycles for thirty-plus years, there can be a sense of something missing from our lives. Where is that old Moon clock, we wonder? The blessed Moon is still your clock, even though you're no longer bleeding. Fall into her rhythm, and listen to her ebb and flow.

I believe the Wise Crone should be acknowledged and celebrated. Our body may not be what it was, now that it has more lines, and there's a stretchiness to our skin, and silver hair. There's another sort of beauty that can come to the Crone if she's been conscious of her lifestyle choices, such as those of nutrition, mindfulness, exercise, and positive thinking. She learns that you're never too old to dance or have a skip in your step! Our 'wise' blood is still inside us. This gives us a wholly new level of wisdom that is ours for the keeping.

Allow at least a couple of hours for the ceremony. Beforehand, the celebrant should ask the Crone to bring something from her life to represent what she is leaving behind. She could write down what this means to her, and attach it to the object.

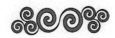

Ask her to look around Mother Nature, and find an item that represents the new life she is walking into. She will bring this with her, too. Again, she can write down what this means to her.

Create a Red Tent. This can be in a living room, or literally within a tent or yurt. It can be in a garden or a clearing in woodland, or on a beach with a circle marked out by seashells.

First, clear the space using sage or lavender. Place symbols on the altar: stars, flowers, cloak, ribbons, gourds. Light black candles. Begin by calling in the ancestresses and Goddesses.

The ceremony is an opportunity for friends to honour the Crone with blessings, songs, stories, poetry, gifts, a foot massage, or head garland. If there are gifts for the Crone, share them now.

As with any ritual and ceremony, there is a basic structure: welcome/introduction, songs, chants, prayers, symbols, rituals, closing. You might like to use the songs mentioned in the section on menarche. Ideally, you will have a celebrant (this needn't be a professional) to guide everyone easily through the ceremony.

Towards the end of the ceremony, the Crone is invited through the passageway. The passage can be a threshold, curtain, gateway, women's arms, or a walkway created from flowers or shells or pine cones.

As a celebrant, it is always worth sharing the significance of this celebration, especially as there are likely to be people in attendance who are unfamiliar with such a ceremony.

When the Crone has walked through the passageway, she can be anointed by the celebrant with lavender or rose oil.

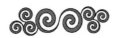

The celebrant asks the Crone if she is ready for her new commitments, and if the Crone is ready to celebrate life as a wise woman. She then places a black cloak around her shoulders, and a crone staff in her hand. If a flower garland or crown has been made, she can wear it as she walks out. The Crone can share her gratitude and her wisdom. This is her chance to inspire those who have yet to walk this path. She then invites her witnesses to join her for a meal.

Sepia and Starflower

There are many wise and wonderful allies from the natural world which can support you across the threshold of menopause and into the world beyond of Crone. My two favourites are sepia and starflower.

Sepia is a homeopathic remedy. In some ways, it reminds me of the Crone's cape! It is the energetic imprint of the ink of the cuttlefish, and is secreted to hide from predators. During menopause (this is often a useful remedy for PMT, too), there may be many times that we wish to go inwards to process our journey, and to appear 'invisible' to the outside world. The keynotes of the sepia remedy include those women who love thunderstorms, and feel better for exercise, such as dancing.

Starflowers grow readily in any garden. Otherwise known as borage, these beautiful flowers are a wonderful support to the adrenal glands. Sip one or two cups of this tea each day.

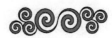

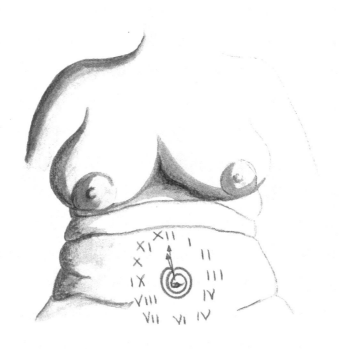

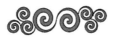

Your cycle is changing. It may be irregular. Describe the letting go process.

Your last blood has flowed. What does this mean for you? How is your life opening up in new ways?

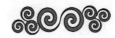

You have an adult lifetime of experience with the flow of red blood. What gifts will you give to your granddaughters, nieces or younger sisters? What gifts would you like to see go into the Red Box of a young maiden? What do you wish for her? What have you learnt? What would you do differently? Create a Crone Box or Basket, and invite women to join your Medicine Wheel ceremony. Ask your guests to bring a nurturing item to include. Afterwards, write down what this experience has meant to you. If this ritual was widespread in our culture, how might our views of older women change?

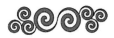

Create a garden of red (menstrual blood) or white (Grandmother Moon) flowers. Maybe you'd like black flowers, such as tulips, to honour the Crone. Or why not mix all three colours for the Menstrual Trinity.

Allow yourself to stand, barefoot, in front of this floral, life-giving altar. You can do this every day, or perhaps you'd prefer to do so at New and Full Moons.

Breathe in the fresh air around you. Hold hands with Mother Earth. You and she are one. The lunar pulse still exists within you long after the last blood has flowed from your body. Allow yourself to connect with the Earth and connect with the Moon. You are a child of the Universe. Thank you.

Dear Crone,
Blessed Be, and Blessed Do.

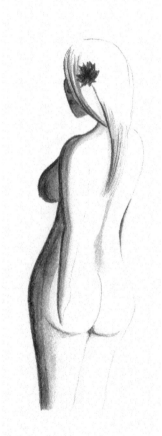

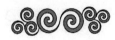

Resource Directory

http://.www.redtentwomensproject.org/
The Red Tent Women's Project is a diverse and dynamic community of women who are catalysts for social change. By creating safe and empowered spaces we facilitate community building, information and resource exchange, and personal growth for women and girls.

http://redtentdirectory.com
http://redtenttemplemovement.com
http://www.redtentwellness.com/index.php
http://www.redtentsisters.com

http://menstruationresearch.org/2012/11/28/occupy-your-period
http://www.jewelswingfield.com/red-tent-circles.php
http://alisastarkweather.com

http://www.femininewear.co.uk
We sell cloth menstrual pads, an alternative to disposable pads and many different brands of menstrual cup. Menstrual cups are made from silicone, latex or plastic. They are a reusable, safe, alternative to tampons. All of our menstrual products are reusable - just right for the eco-conscious consumer.

http://www.newmoonpads.com
Beautiful cloth pads. One new moon pad = 100 – 150 disposable pads
http://www.newmoonpads.com/themonthly.html Periodical about menstruation

http://lunapads.com
http://www.womensquest.org

Red Tent Bournemouth, Dorset, UK

This is a safe, sacred, and transformative space for women. Red Tent Bournemouth is a collaboration of women – we have almost 200 women in our community, and this is expanding all the time. This space is open to all women who have ever menstruated. We have a beautiful monthly gathering, we run regular workshops and retreats (including our two-day 'Journey Into The Sacred Feminine' retreat), and we provide a sacred space for pregnant women. We hold space for women to explore birth trauma, and the mother wound. And we provide holistic support and guidance around menopause. Contact us about our 'Moon-Girl Warriors', a powerful coming-of-age program for nine to 12-year-old girls. This includes an eight-week Rite-Of-Passage Mentorship program for girls. Red Tent Bournemouth also provides women with a huge variety of resources and information for all stages of life and aspects of womanhood. For further information please contact: Teresa Bilowus 07501322294 Helen Gialias 07825447756 Email: redtentbournemouth@ gmail.com Facebook Open Group: Red Tent Bournemouth

Not Just a Piece of Cloth

www.njpc.goonj.org Barely 12%of India's menstruating women use pads.

Around 70% of women in India say their family can't afford to buy pads. Goonj (means *an echo*), a multi award-winning social enterprise, started the NJPC (Not Just a Piece of Cloth) initiative in 2005. NJPC is focused on opening up the most taboo and ignored subject of menstrual hygiene: a female health hazard, by involving the masses in generating an affordable cloth napkin. The NJPC programme is a nationwide intervention, which not only starts with providing a physical product but stresses more on changing practices, behavioural patterns, education and replication in the long term. *My Pad*, Goonj's clean cloth pad, is developed out of old cloth collected from urban masses. It is made with highly indigenous processes while also educating the user women to make it on their own. NJPC - *A Million Voices* campaign and website is initiated by Goonj, and is an extension of its ongoing work across India. Our aim is to spread global awareness about this basic need and get more people to talk about it, to break the taboo and shame around this natural process.

Museum of Menstruation
www.mum.org

http://www.moonsong.com.au/
Welcome to Moonsong, a website for women. Reclaiming feminine power through reconnection with the women's mysteries. The women's mysteries are: the shamanic journeys of our rites of passage of menarche, childbirth, and menopause; the spiritual practice of menstruation; the inner, spiritual and shamanic journey of pregnancy, birth and mothering; and menopause as rebirth. The information within Moonsong will help the healing of the wounded feminine and reawaken feminine power for the benefit of all. You will find information and tools for menstruation, childbirth, connecting with the cycles and passing on this wisdom to our children.

http://www.mirandagray.co.uk/
Author of Red Moon

http://laraowen.com/
Author of Her Blood is Gold

www.redwisdom.co.uk

Eco Rainbow
www.ecorainbow.co.uk/
Eco-friendly alternatives to disposable menstrual pads.

www.moontimes.co.uk
We stock fair-trade organic cloth pads, wool pads, moon sponges and cups, cycle charting and wise woman books, Moon Maiden Menarche gift sets, postpartum pad sets, and new mother gifts sets, and lots more! Rachael Hertogs is the author of *Menarche: a Journey into Womanhood*. Moon Times menstrual products are used by all women of all ages, all over the world! Washable organic & patterned cloth pads & panty liners, Moon sponges &

cups are becoming more and more popular; they are the comfortable & safe alternatives to disposables; free from bleaches, irritants and chemicals! We also stock many other products for the green-minded woman! Many of our products will last for years and save you £100s; being kind to your purse whilst being kind to the planet! Reusable menstrual products are safer for your body and more cost effective; they are not a step back in time but a positive step towards our planet's well-being! Our products are an alternative to 'disposable' sanitary products and are ideal gifts for: young women new to their menses, new mothers who need soft cloth against their delicate tissue after giving birth, women who suffer from slight incontinence. At Moon Times, we empower women in body appreciation, environmental awareness, and self-respect through the use of eco-menstrual products.

Red Wisdom was founded by Karin Chandler to support women and girls to embrace the journey of womanhood through women's circles, workshops and campaigning. It promotes women's right to live in a world where our womb-bleeding is not seen as dirty or shaming, but as a natural and healthy process. It helps women to value their bleeding, seeing it as a sacred tool and part of a bigger template which links into the energies of Sun, Moon, land, sea and sky.

A menstrual activist, workshop facilitator and apprentice wise woman, Karin works with both a political and a Pagan spiritual thread. She runs workshops exploring the mandala of the menstrual cycle, enabling mothers to prepare their daughters for menarche, ceremonies for adult women to reclaim their menarche, and women's circles to enable women to share their stories. Workshops are run at camps, festivals and from the Red Wisdom Hearth (in Skenfrith, S.E. Wales). She also blogs regularly about menstruation and other issues which relate to the stages of womanhood. You can read her blogs and find out more at www.redwisdom.co.uk and on the Facebook page Red Wisdom Hearth.

CD
Blessingway Songs CD by Copperwoman
http://www.copperwoman.com/pages/music.html
www.blessingwaysongs.org This CD is perfect for Blessingways, but also has songs suitable for various Red Tent activities. Beware, the songs are catchy!

Jewellery
Wild Mother Arts http://www.wildmotherarts.com

Red hemp thread
http://hemphutt.com/coloredhemp.html

Candles
http://www.stevalcandlecompany.co.uk/
http://www.beeswaxco.com/
http://www.queenb.com.au/

Mandala prints to purchase for the altar
http://themandalajourney.com/store/prints/

Finger labyrinths and more
www.ispiritual.com/
www.fingerlabyrinths.com/
www.madmoonarts.com
www.sevenstonespottery.com

Healing Orchids (for flower, plant and gem essences)
Achamore House, Isle of Gigha, Argyll, Scotland PA41 7AD
www.healingorchids.com Tel: 01 583 505 385

Earth Paint   http://www.naturalearthpaint.com/

Recommended Books

Bennett, J. (2002) A Blessing not a Curse: A mother daughter guide to the transition from child to woman, Sally Milner Publishing, Bowral, 2002.

Bennett, J. & Naish F. (2004)The Natural Fertility Management Contraception and Conception Kits

Diamant, A. (2002). The Red Tent. London: Pan Books.

Northrup, Christiane Dr. (1998) Women's Bodies, Women's Wisdom. New York: Bantam Books.

Owen, L. (2008). Her Blood is Gold. Dorset: Archive Publishing.

Pope, A. (2001). The Wild Genie: the healing power of menstruation. Bowral, Australia: Sally Milner Publishing. (out of print, second hand copies may be available on the web)

Richardson, D. Tantric Orgasm for Women, Destiny Books, Rochester, 2004. (Diana's website: www.livinglove.com)

Singer, K. (2004). The Garden of Fertility: A Guide to Charting Your Fertility Signals to Prevent or Achieve Pregnancy (Naturally)and to Gauge Your Reproductive Health. New York: Avery

Weed, S. New Menopausal Years: The Wise Woman W – Alternative Approaches for Women 30–90

Weschler, T. (2001) Taking Charge of Your Fertility

http://thehappywomb.com
Reaching for the Moon - a girl's guide to her female cycles
By Lucy Pearce
82 pages. (June 2013)
ISBN: 1482363038
Written for girls aged 9-14 introducing them to the menstrual cycle in simple, soulful language, taking the form of a gentle, meaningful initiation into womanhood. Reaching for the Moon incorporates stories, real women's experiences of their first periods, and answers girls' most burning questions about periods and their bodies in a loving, age-appropriate way. This is the guide that empowered and caring mothers, aunts and godmothers want for the girls in their lives.

Moon Time: a guide to celebrating your menstrual cycle
By Lucy Pearce
144 pages. (February 2012)
ISBN: 1468056719

A guide for all menstrual women from 14- 40. Referred to by readers world wide as "life changing". Moon Time will help you to embrace all aspects of your menstrual cycle, heal PMS, develop self-care practices, and reconnect to your body's natural rhythms. It is the first book in print to explore the new phenomenon of red tents as places for women's retreat, and shares how to create a red tent for yourself and your community, as well as how to celebrate a girl's transition to womanhood.

About the author

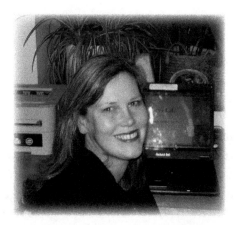

Veronika Sophia Robinson was born and raised in South East Queensland, Australia, the fourth of eight children, and enjoyed living in the great Australian bush amongst the eucalyptus trees, red soil, continuous sunshine, and kangaroos.

At 23, she moved to New Zealand, later meeting the love of her life and having two gorgeous daughters.

Veronika is the author of many non-fiction books which cover natural parenting, holistic health, and good plant-based cooking. She is also a children's writer, novelist, and a journalist. She has been a celebrant since 1995, when she began officiating wedding ceremonies in New Zealand. She has also been a celebrant for the following ceremonies: house blessing; divorce; menarche; menopause; baby naming; Handfasting, Blessingway; letting go; Phoenix.

Her passions include being a wife and mother, metaphysics and spirituality, psychological astrology, walking, vegetarian cooking, organic gardening by the Moon, living in accord with Nature, writing and music.

Veronika lives with her family in a 300-year-old sandstone cottage overlooking fields and fells in rural Cumbria in the north of England. Veronika is available for mother-to-mother mentoring, astrological consultations and to facilitate women's workshops. www.veronikarobinson.com

About the artist

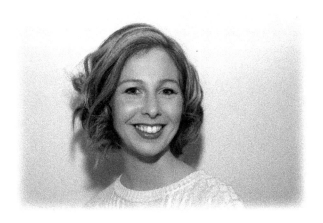

For Susan this book came at the perfect time in her life. A mother with a passion for women's rights and birth rights, Susan has been on a journey of discovery. This journey through her own births, and supporting the births of others as a doula, has led her back to art. Embracing now the fabulous world of art and illustration, Susan is inspired by strength, femininity, passion, motherhood and political struggle. *Cycle to the Moon* has given Susan the space to entwine her passions of feminism and art; symbolic of her own journey back to the feminine.

Find more of Susan's work at susanmerrick.co.uk or chat with her on Facebook
https://m.facebook.com/SbmArtwork
Or twitter.
https://mobile.twitter.com/smdoula
Some of Susan's work is available as beautiful Giclee prints here
https://www.etsy.com/shop/SBMArtwork

Artwork from *Cycle to the Moon* is available from Susan's website to purchase as prints.
www.susanmerrick.co.uk

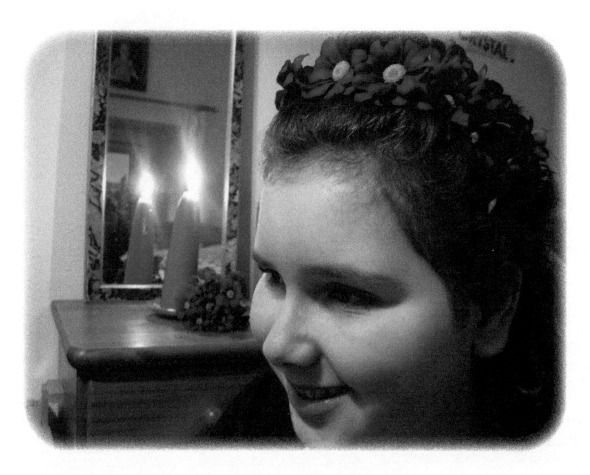

My beautiful young Maiden, celebrating menarche.

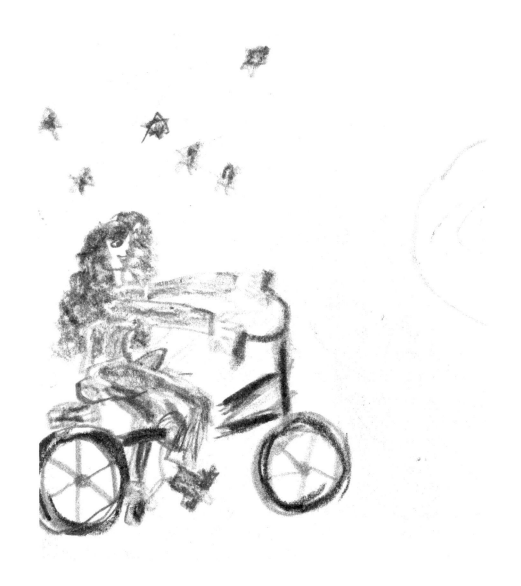

A special thank you to my daughter, Bethany, who drew me this cover
for Cycle to the Moon when she was a young girl.

About the publisher

Starflower Press is a boutique publisher with a focus on conscious parenting, health, holistic living, as well as Young Adult fiction, illustrated children's books, and novels. www.starflowerpress.com

Starflower Press draws its name and inspiration from the olden-day herb, Borage (Borago Officinalis). It is still found in many places, though is often thought of as a wild flower, rather than a herb. Starflower is recognisable by its beautiful star-like flowers, which are formed by five petals of intense blue (sometimes it is pink). The unusual blue colour was used in Renaissance paintings. The Biblical meaning of this blue is heavenly grace. Borage, from the Celt borrach, means courage. Throughout history, Starflower has been associated with courage.

To find more of our publications, visit: www.starflowerpress.com

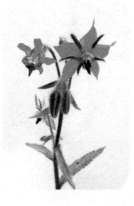

Notes

Lightning Source UK Ltd.
Milton Keynes UK
UKHW052344010720
365828UK00006B/119